Foods For

Fabulous

Sex

D1373629

By Dr. Morton Walker

Natural Sexual Nutrients to Trigger Passion,
Heighten Response, Improve Performance, and
Overcome Dysfunction

Foods For Fabulous Sex

Copyright © 1992
By Dr. Morton Walker

Published in the United States By
The Magni Group, Inc.
P.O. Box 849
McKinney, Texas 75070

Manufactured in the United States of America

ISBN 1-882330-20-X

About the Author

Dr. Morton Walker having left almost 17 years of doctoral practice in 1969, has since worked full time as a professional freelance medical journalist. His special areas of interest are improvements in human sexuality, loving relationships, and better sex.

The author of 53 books and over 1400 magazine, newspaper, and clinical journal articles, Dr. Walker has presented or appeared on more than 900 media events. These have included national, international (by satellite) and local radio and television talk shows, press interviews, lectures, videofilms, audiotapes, and news conferences.

Disclaimer

This book has been written and published strictly for informational purposes, and should not be used as a substitute for your own health care professional's advice.

The author, Dr. Morton Walker is a professional medical journalist reporting on such nutritional, sexual, illness, and health information as has been included in this book.

You should not consider educational material published here to be the practice of medicine, sexology, nutrition, dietetics, psychology, or the rendering of any other form of health care. Almost all the facts and other information written here by Dr. Walker have come from the files, publications, and personal interviews of informed doctors who diagnose and treat with holistic methods and/or their patients who have suffered from problems of sexual deterioration. Moreover, clinical journal articles, popular magazine articles, material from published books, lecture presentations, audiotapes, case reports, anecdotes, testimonials, patient histories, and other information have been utilized to educate interested readers.

If you or your acquaintance, as a potential user of knowledge received from these pages, require opinions, diagnoses, treatments, therapeutic advice, correction of lifestyle, or any other aid relating to sexual or nutritional illness or wellness, it is recommended that you or your acquaintance consult either health care professionals who have contributed to this book, or your own medical expert on the chronic signs and symptoms of altered sexuality that one may face.

Please be mindful that the author in no way takes responsibility for the expertise, skills, knowledge, training, honesty, integrity, diagnostic abilities, treatment procedures, or other acumen of the physicians listed therein. Dr. Walker accepts no liability for acts of commission or omission by these doctors.

The statements you are reading should be considered disclaimers of responsibility for anything published in this book. As the author, Dr. Walker and the publisher are providing information with the understanding that you may act on it at your own risk and also with full awareness that health professionals should first be consulted. Their specific advice for you or your acquaintance should be considered before using anything that you read here.

Table of Contents

Prologue

Have you reached the point in life where sex is no longer as exciting, as interesting or as frequent as it used to be?

Is your sexual urge of earlier years lost but not forgotten?

Are you wondering if there are products that might again turn you on sexually, if only you knew what to use?

Do you have sexual fantasies?

Are you feeling apathetic about lovemaking but you wish you could be ignited to a livelier sexual response?

Has the bedroom activity (or non-activity) with your spouse deteriorated so that dissatisfaction has set in for both of you?

Does a particular sexual dysfunction cause you to shun, either consciously or unconsciously, the usual male-female relationship?

If you answered "Yes" to any one of these questions, please realize that you are not alone. A lot of others affirm sexual inadequacy in their lives. In a study published in the *New England Journal of Medicine* involving "happily married" couples, 63 percent of the women reported having difficulty getting sexually excited and reaching orgasm. A full 70 percent of the responding men admitted to erection and ejaculation failure. In addition, lack of desire and the inability to relax and enjoy the sex act were defined as problems by 77 percent of the women and 50 percent of the men. The report was surprising, as the doctors doing the research

7

pointed out that these were couples well established as sex partners. Consider how much more unhappiness might have been reported if the study had been carried out among single men and women.

Sex counselors from all over the world, reporting in other current medical journals, give additional statistics on eight different forms of sexual hang-ups, inhibitions, incapacity, and lack of libido (sex drive). Over half of all men and women in Western industrialized society have problems with their sexuality today. These sexologists claim that virtually every man and woman will, at some time, experience at least one episode of impotence or frigidity (lack of sexual feeling or response).

Yet, no other activity—directly or indirectly—so dominates our thoughts or lives than the pursuit of sexual fulfillment. People are more preoccupied than ever with sex. If you add up all the radio songs, television stories, films, plays, magazine pieces, newspaper articles, and books revolving around sex and love, you will see how important human sexuality has become. The era of altered sexual conventions is upon us. The etiquette of sex has become more open and liberal. Today, we are no longer supposed to suppress our natural sexual inclinations as we did at the beginning of the 20th century.

This change in how our culture regards sexual expression came about with Sigmund Freud, in the mid-1900s. The father of modern psychoanalysis first expanded our concept of sexuality to the "seeking of pleasure" rather than solely for reproduction. He introduced us to our libidos.

While Freud pointed out that sexual needs are instinctive, he never found a definitive solution for why all of us don't have great sex lives. Even now, no sex counselor using Freudian concepts ever blames the patient's physical self. Emphasis is placed strictly on that important sex organ between one's two ears—the brain. The truth of this statement was brought home to me in Chicago, in June 1983, when I appeared on *Kup's Show,* a television panel program, with celebrity sex counselor Ruth Westheimer, Ph.D., adjunct associate professor in the department of psychiatry at The New York Hospital-Cornell Medical Center. I saw her eyes light up with a "eureka experience" (a revolutionary thought) when I presented proof that a lackluster sex life (or even a good one that should be great) may be caused by deficiencies in a person's diet. After we videotaped the show, Dr. Westheimer wrote down the names and dosages of many nutrients I had discussed before the television cameras.

Most of us never live up to the idealized portraits of sexuality that we see and hear every day through the electronic media and in the press. We all spend thousands of dollars each year on clothes, cosmetics, deodorants, perfumes, and other items to make us more attractive to the opposite sex. However, we rarely give any thought to how our sex organs work and what we can do to help them give us greater heights of physical pleasure. Isn't it logical that a good sex performance isn't something that just happens but rather has to be worked at, nurtured, and protected? Nevertheless, too many of us are ignorant of what our bodies are trying to tell us when our sexual apparatus does not work well.

Surveys among physicians show that the average doctor receives three complaints a week from patients suffering from some sexual malady.

Leading sexologists Masters and Johnson have gone so far as to conclude that at least 50 percent of all marriages in the United States are plagued with some form of sexual inadequacy, which confirms what sex counselors around the world have reported in medical journals. Statistics indicate a wide variance in the frequency of lovemaking among married people, which is more closely related to the amount of free time the couple has, rather than their innate desire for sexual contact. One study, published in *Medical Aspects of Human Sexuality*, found that a large group of couples in their 30s, at the height of their sexual inclinations, averaged only 7.78 acts of coitus per month. Another group, between 40 and 50 years of age, averaged coital incidence of just 6.98 times per month. By age 60 to 70, the amount of coital contact had declined to once a week or less.

Fortunately, 25 years' exploration by Freudian psychiatrists into the whys and wherefores of human sexual response has coincided with 25 years of intense investigation by orthomolecular psychiatrists into Americans' nutritional needs. A comparison of the two investigations sheds new light on what people need to do to live at peak sexual power from puberty to the day of death.

Chapter 1

Nutritional Aphrodisiacs

Sexologists who use nutrition as part of their treatment (a rare breed of health professionals) know that there is nothing magical about igniting sexual passion or overcoming sexual dysfunction. Instead, they have pinpointed the pleasure-making neural pathways in the brain and followed their biochemical impulses all the way to the sex act itself. Rather than sexual arousal being only a matter of the right time, right place, and right person, now we know that it is also a matter of correct biochemistry, hormones present when they're needed, and the appropriate nutrients to act as energizers, metabolizers, stimulators, free radical scavengers, antioxidants, co-enzymes, and mood elevators.

What are these substances that create heightened sexual desire, positive response to sexual advances, and enhancement of the gonads? They are natural nutritional aphrodisiacs available to almost everyone.

Aphrodisiac, a singular potion that heightens the sexual urge and promotes amorous intentions, derives from Aphrodite, the Greek goddess of love. Some "aphrodisiacs" do work—and some don't.

Here you will learn the truth about authentic sexual stimuli and those only alleged to be.

For centuries men and women have been employing certain substances to increase sexual potency by stimulating the sex glands or working directly on the sex organs. Often greatly exaggerated, reports on their effectiveness have been passed along from person to person almost as long as civilization has existed. Today, we substitute other objects for aphrodisiacs. "Sex aids" such as peek-a-boo nightgowns and frilly, revealing underwear are very much in demand at department stores. Certain colognes are supposed to help stimulate the sexual imagination. People pay through the nose, thinking that they are buying better sex. When a British Sterling™ cologne television advertisement featured a sexy woman whispering, "My men wear British Sterling or they wear nothing at all," sales skyrocketed.

Actually, the mind exerts such a powerful influence over your sexual self that just about anything can work as an aphrodisiac if you believe in it. Some people swear by powdered rhinoceros horn, which is ineffective, expensive, and hard to find. So-called aphrodisiacs such as Spanish Fly often contain overly caustic and dangerous chemicals. Spanish Fly is derived from the insect *Lytta vesicatoria*, a shiny green and gold beetle, known to Greeks and Romans as *Cantharides*. Made into candies and cakes for private parties, Cantharides finds a small but steady market in the Arab countries. As a caustic taken internally, it irritates the genitalia which become stimulated by the irritation, and sexual desires have been known to increase accordingly. The stuff brings on bloody discharges from the kidneys and death from overdoses can occur. The only legitimate use of

Spanish Fly is in veterinary medicine: given to bulls for stud purposes.

Speaking of bulls, prairie oysters are the Midwestern version of a natural aphrodisiac. These regional delicacies are actually bull testicles, and Texas macho-types claim that eating prairie oysters can make a man incredibly potent. The bull testicles apparently contain a great deal of protein in the form of concentrated glandular substances that can have human testicles functioning exactly like the bull's. No doubt there is some nourishment derived from consuming prairie oysters; they could probably be classified as a nutritional aphrodisiac.

Red wine is supposed to promote relaxation and a lessening of sexual inhibitions. This belief may be bona fide, because red wine causes the body to produce histamines. Experiments by pharmaceutical companies indicate that histamines can shorten the time it takes to reach orgasm and can intensify the experience. For good scientific reasons, women benefit from drinking red wine more than men.

Carl C. Pfeiffer, M.D., Ph.D., former medical director of the Brain Bio Center of Princeton, New Jersey, found that the histamine levels of women—and therefore, their orgasm capacity—can be raised by taking the B-complex vitamin pantothenic acid and the bioflavonoid rutin, a substance related to vitamin C. Dr. Pfeiffer explained, "Low histamine females have historically been labeled as frigid. We now know, however, that the female with high histamine levels may have repeated orgasms or highly sustained orgasms."

Some women who previously experienced difficulty climaxing, followed the Pfeiffer nutritional program and discovered that they could now fully achieve this special pleasure. Others

13

found that the time it took to climax was shortened or that the number of orgasms was increased.

The vitamins pantothenic acid and rutin may be swallowed as supplements in pill form or eaten in foods in which they have higher concentrations. These vitamins may help the pre-orgasmic woman finally come to climax during sexual intercourse.

A few foods with high quantities of pantothenic acid are **brewers yeast, liver, peanuts, mushrooms, peas, eggs, oatmeal, torula yeast, soybeans, perch, pecans, garbanzos, kale, cauliflower, sardines, avocados, sunflower seeds, lentils, whole wheat, brown rice, and salmon.**

Foods with large quantities of rutin are **grapes, all citrus fruit, cherries, parsley, cabbage, peppers, all tropical fruit, melons, rose hips, prunes, plums, apricots, blackberries, black currants, and broccoli.**

Although drinking red wine is not disadvantageous to sexuality, overindulging in hard liquor does not mix well with romance. Alcoholic beverages may relax a person enough to be more willing, but they also lower blood sugar levels so fast that seldom will you have the energy to finish what you've begun. While whisky, vodka, gin and brandy may be all right in moderation for a woman, they play havoc with men, in whom over-imbibing can cause temporary impotence.

Herbal Aphrodisiacs

An African herb, yohimbe, has traditionally been used to fuel sexual desire and receptivity. And another herb, kavakava, from the islands of the South Pacific, is brewed into a tea to stimulate sexuality. Both herbs affect the central nervous system in the same way the conglomeration of sexual feelings, emotions, and visual and tactile stimuli work on the body. The plant damiana, found in the West Indies, Mexico, and the American Southwest, is used by knowledgeable lovers to bring on more prolonged intimacy. These three herbs may be considered nutritional aphrodisiacs, inasmuch as they are metabolized in the body, but possible side effects mean that precautions should be taken if they are used.

Yohimbe, *Corynanthe yohimbini*, had been touted as an effective remedy for human impotence ever since black Africans were brought as slaves to the New World. They carried the knowledge with them. Veterinarians have utilized this remedy, too, to stimulate lazy bulls and stallions. Yohimbe is extracted as a white powder from the Indian snakeroot *Rauwolfia serpentina*. Yohimbe is actually a drug. It penetrates the blood-brain barrier to produce increased pulse, sweating, physical restlessness, urine retention, and an elevation of blood pressure. It causes a mild psychedelic effect by blocking the neurotransmitters, acetylcholine and epinephrine, when it is taken in doses above 50 milligrams (mg). There is a heightening of skin sensitivity. Some aphrodisia may come from its inhibition of serotonin, a vasoconstrictor, and of monoamine oxidase (MAO), the enzyme that ordinarily protects you against amines, which cause blood pressure fluctuations. Yohimbe should not be taken with sedatives, antihistamines, amphetamines, diet pills, alcohol, cocoa, pineapples, bananas, and other foods rich in amino acid tyrosin. People suffering from diabetes, hypoglycemia, liver disease, heart disease, kidney disease, or peripheral vascular disease should avoid its use. Following is the recipe for yohimbe cocktail:

> **Yohimbe Cocktail**
>
> **Simmer 3 to 6 teaspoons of yohimbe (purchased from an herbologist or herb shop) in a pint of water for 10 minutes. Start with a small dose if you've never used it or you are of low body weight. As the tea cools, dissolve 1000 mg of vitamin C in the cup and sip the brew. Honey may be added for flavoring.**

In this form, the yohimbi ascorbate in the low dosage you're taking is nutritious and the only way yohimbe should be used. Make sure your sex partner is nearby as you get turned on.

When yohimbe is combined with hydrochloric acid in a standardized dosage, a psychedelic sensation occurs when the compound is swallowed or sniffed. This is yohimbine hydrochloride, an adrenergic blocking agent that alters the brain's mood. No way is yohimbine hydrochloride a nutritional product. It is strictly a drug, not recommended for use.

Kavakava, *Piper methysticum*, mainly affects the spinal nerves to produce an ecstatic warmth by flooding the genitals with blood. Its only problem is that it causes drowsiness within an hour or so of ingestion. When the kavakava liquid is placed on the glans penis or clitoris, mild tingling of the nerve endings provides a slow buildup of charge in the deeper fibers before orgasm. For a man who regularly experiences premature ejaculation, kavakava oil patted onto his erect penis will afford him more relaxed control. His ejaculatory response will be slower, so that he may last longer during vaginal penetration. Following is the recipe for a kavakava drink:

Kavakava Drink

Take 1 ounce of chopped or ground herb and mix it in a blender with 2 tablespoons of coconut oil (or other food oil). Add 1 tablespoon of lecithin granules or powder, and a cup or more of purified water, coconut milk, or skimmed milk, plus chopped ice. Before drinking, strain the fluid. Depending on how much liquid you add, this drink will make from 2 to 4 servings for a sexy good time. You can also freeze the drink into ice cubes for future sexual indulgence, but the fresh solution seems to have a more powerful effect on the genitals.

Damiana, *Turnera aphriodisiaca*, is well respected among Mexicans and Brazilians as a palliative and tonic for correcting male erectile difficulties. Chemically related to the poison strychnine, damiana acts in a similar manner, but is much safer. It sends messages along the nerves in all directions. Livestock breeders use the herb to stimulate their studs. A Philadelphia physician, W. H. Myers, M.D., after giving his impotent patients 15 to 30 drops of damiana extract per day, reported that damiana is "the most effective and only remedy that in my hands had a successful result in all cases."

Women who drank damiana tea before bedtime told of having highly erotic dreams. Drinking the beverage over a period of time has a cumulative effect. Women report that they become progressively more sensitive to oral, manual or penile stimulation of the clitoris. Following is the recipe for damiana tea:

Damiana Tea

Simmer 2 tablespoons of the dried herb in a large cup of hot water in an infuser for 5 minutes. Then slowly sip the brew.

No more than a cup of damiana tea daily is recommended, since too much of the brew may cause liver problems.

There is also a damiana drink you can mix and enjoy as a sexy nightcap, especially served chilled, in a cordial glass. According to Adam Gottlieb, author of *Sex Drugs and Aphrodisiacs*:

Damiana Drink

Soak one ounce of dried damiana in a pint of vodka for 5 days. Filter the liquid well. Then, again soak the leaves for 5 days, but this time use purified water (avoid chlorinated water). Filter this solution. Warm the water extract to not more than 150° F and mix with 3/4 cup of honey. Then, combine the water extract and vodka extract. Chill.

The result is a fine cocktail for you and your sexmate. I recommend only one ounce of this mixture for its aphrodisiac quality; that way, you will imbibe only one-half ounce of liquor. Rather than storing the remainder as ice cubes, let the damiana drink age in a decanter for a few weeks in the refrigerator and enjoy it when desired.

In Brazil, the natives consider beverages made from damiana leaves nutritional tonics. They drink them for the slow build-up of aphrodisiac effect and as therapeutic agents for the kidneys.

Herbal remedies for reduced libido are among the oldest known medical preparations. While they don't claim miracles, herbal tonics and teas definitely have been shown to restore sexual interest for both men and women.

Foremost among the latter day sexual rejuvenators is the herb ginseng. Used in the Orient as a general body tonic for several centuries, ginseng has recently been scrutinized by scientists to see why it benefits sexual response and performance.   They found that because it strengthens and stimulates the endocrine glands, ginseng has a profound effect on the output of sex hormones.   The medical director of the Largo Center of Preventive and General Medicine of Largo, Florida, Donald J. Carrow, M.D., medical consultant to the Institute of Sexual Research in Ft. Lauderdale, Florida, has a high regard for ginseng as a sexual energizer.   He credits it with increasing libido, potency, and vigor.

Ground ginseng powder for brewing into tea may be purchased by mail order from herbal supply houses or from herb shops.

Thus, aphrodisiacs taken specifically to enhance sexual pleasure, correct sexual dysfunction, increase libido, or experience erotic dreaming may be for the purpose of excitement, arousal, nourishment, intoxication, or just plain fun.   Most have a short term effect.   They work quickly and fade quickly.   You should be more interested in those nutritional aphrodisiacs that work over the long term—such as ginseng.   A premenopausal or postmenopausal woman taking doses of ginseng daily probably will avoid having the discomforting symptoms of life change such as flushes.   Because ginseng is a stabilizer of the body systems, with special affinity for the gonads, it catalyzes the sex organs into functioning, when the command comes from your brain.

Ginseng is typical of dozens of nutritional aphrodisiacs—oral sex products I call "nutridisiacs"—which comprise genuine dietary ingredients.   The pantothenic acid and rutin described earlier are fine examples of nutridisiacs. Taking them regularly as part of your diet strengthens your sex organs and makes your nervous system more sensitive to pleasurable sensations. If you're looking for renewed sexual vigor, relief from impotency, revitalization of sexual enthusiasm, restoration of lost orgasms (or discovery of orgasm you never had), return of ejaculation ability, and a surge of sexual energy, read on about nutridisiacs. They trigger primal sexual response.

Sexual Help from Nutridisiacs

Few currently practicing physicians, using strictly traditional allopathic or standard osteopathic methods of treatment, know anything about nutridisiacs. The truth is that most medical doctors (M.D.s) or doctors of osteopathy (D.O.s) are not trained in nutritional therapy techniques. Of 143 medical schools in the United States and Canada, for instance, only about 15 have required courses in clinical nutrition.

Sohrab Mobarhan, M.D., a gastroenterologist at the University of Illinois College of Medicine, pointed out the problem during an interview. Dr. Mobarhan admitted that "Medical schools tended to overlook nutrition until recently because it was assumed that if a person lived in a wealthy country and had enough money to buy food, he would not have a nutritional problem. Now that attitude is beginning to change because research has shown that 40 percent of all patients who are hospitalized are malnourished."

Mildred S. Seelig, M.D., Ph.D., and expert on magnesium metabolism and editor of the *Journal of the American College of Nutrition*, said: "The amounts of time and attention devoted to nutrition vary from school to school. It is still possible for medical students to get almost no training in nutrition except for what they are taught in biochemistry about acute nutritional states such as beriberi. The crucial factor is the attitude of the faculty. Some departmental chairmen don't want nutrition taught today because they didn't have a course when they were students and so they don't believe nutrition is important."

Myron Winick, M.D., director of the Institute of Human Nutrition at Columbia-Presbyterian Medical Center in New York City, further explained the lack of medical nutrition knowledge among doctors. He said, "It has been difficult for medical schools to find a home for nutrition in the curriculum because no one department is responsible for teaching it. This wasn't true at the beginning of this century because nutrition was what biochemistry was all about. However, after the Second World War, molecular biology came to the forefront of biochemistry and nutrition got overlooked."

In the past, nutrition and sexuality were seldom covered in the medical-school curriculum. The doctors considered nutrition and sexuality just fads; such fads, they believed, would not last and there was no reason to waste time educating patients about them. Today, however, the consumer insists on his or her "right to know," and clinicians have had to take heed of their patients' demands. Consequently, in some cases, nutrition and sexuality are being added to school curriculums as faculty members are recognizing that such knowledge will enable physicians to relate better to their patients. The inquiring medical consumer is having an effect on medical practitioners.

"It has been very worthwhile," agrees Dr. Winick, "because the commitment [to learning about nutrition and other changes in the practice of medicine] is paying off in better patient care."

However, because sexuality and nutrition are not covered in most medical schools, it's unfair to expect the modern physician to impart such information to patients along these lines. Simply, doctors hardly know much more than an ordinary person who has done some thorough reading on the two subjects.

Further, even less is known about sexual nutrition and, specifically, nutritional aphrodisiacs. Yet, the search for ways to increase sexual desirability, performance, excitement, and response goes back further than recorded history. And today, we unquestionably live in the age of sexual enlightenment. Nutridisiacs can help to bring about the sexual fulfillment desired by so many. Nutridisiacs can truly improve sexual pleasure and capability. Research proves that a number of substances contained in foods, when taken collectively, can almost guarantee you a great sex life by maintaining your body in optimal fitness, complete homeostasis, and peak performance. Having a healthy body is the main requirement. Certain foods definitely have an erotic effect on the user. The best advice for anyone seeking a love charm is to keep one's sexual apparatus working at optimum pitch through the ingestion of nutridisiacs.

Nevertheless, note that nothing in this book substitutes for advice from a physician knowledgeable in nutrition and sexuality. Search out the health professional who can best help you to correct sexual dysfunction. Don't rely only on what is written here.

Heightening Female Orgasm

Sexual orgasm is the natural inheritance of almost everyone. Still, a number of unhappy women label themselves "frigid" because their husbands find them cold, aloof, and disinclined to engage in sexual intercourse. Moreover, the women say they seldom, if ever, experience the ecstatic sensation of orgasm. On one hand, they blame this on their belief that some women are just naturally non-orgasmic; on the other, they say they are too neurotic to climax during coitus. Neither reason has validity, in most cases.

"Frigid" is a cruel term, and, in my opinion, should be abolished when referring to a non-orgasmic or pre-orgasmic woman. The woman who cannot climax may be suffering from the inability to relax during sex. Remember Dr. Carl Pfeiffer's discovery of "low histamine release"? Women with this condition do not release enough histamine during sex. Many researchers now consider histamine the key to orgasmic intensity, frequency, and response. When a woman does not release enough histamine to achieve climax, she becomes frustrated and tense, which further discourages orgasm from taking place. Thus, a vicious non-orgasmic cycle results.

Dr. Pfeiffer and other holistic physicians using therapeutic nutrition who have duplicated his treatment program, have developed a virtual "cure" for low-histamine-caused lack of orgasm. In addition to the use of pantothenic acid and rutin (already described), you should become aware of the beneficial effects of other nutrients for the non-orgasmic or only slightly orgasmic woman.

Niacin (vitamin B-3) can become a most erotic vitamin for women when the overall flush it produces in the body is utilized for sexual advantage. You may have taken niacin (also known as nicotinic acid) in the form of a B-complex tablet or capsule. If your body is not used to the dosage in the single pill that contains niacin alone, you will experience an overall flush, caused by the blood vessels closest to the skin widening and filling with blood, which, in turn, creates a warm, tingling sensation that begins in the ears and neck, moves down into the breasts and upper torso, and eventually extends into the lower abdomen and genital region.

As this very warm and sensual feeling spreads, the skin becomes pinkish, which Masters and Johnson say is a visual signal of primal sexual response. This niacin-induced flush makes the skin feel more alive, more sensitive to the touch, and helps to heighten the physical sensations of sex. If you can time your niacin flush with the onset of orgasm—even if the orgasmic sensation is slight—your feeling will become deeper and longer-lasting.

The average orgasmic woman feels orgasmic contractions at intervals of eight tenths of a second in a series of four or five contractions. Adding niacin to your nutrition may allow you to build up to six seconds in a series of eight contractions. Niacin nutrition can really transport you to the ultimate sexual experience.

It's best to keep the concentration of niacin elevated in your blood continuously rather than merely to pop down niacin pills just before engaging in sexual activity. That way, your body is always capable of more intense orgasms that stay with you for a prolonged time. One highly effective method is to take niacin as a sexual supplement on a continuous basis, 100 mg or more at the end of each meal and 200 mg or more just before slipping into bed with your lover, which should be enough to assure you of a good skin flush.

Another way to keep the blood level of niacin elevated is to eat foods packed with the vitamin. Examples of food containing high concentrations of vitamin B-3 are **rice bran and rice polishings, peanuts, turkey, chicken, trout, halibut, mackerel, swordfish, goose, lamb, sesame seeds, lean beef, pine nuts, buckwheat, barley, split peas, herring, almonds, shrimp, haddock, and veal.**

Another vitamin to help pre-orgasmic women, and those who experience only diminished orgasms, is pyridoxine (vitamin B-6). Pyridoxine will eventually help you climax closer to when your male partner does. Sexologists have established that a woman takes longer to become aroused and reach orgasm than a man. So while a healthy man may be able to climax two or three times during a night of lovemaking, a woman can reach the heights of joy five, six, or more times if she is properly stimulated.

Pyridoxine is reputed to be beneficial for both sexes because it becomes involved in so many metabolic processes. While it has been referred to as the female's necessary nutrient (see the section on pre-menstrual syndrome), pyridoxine also plays an exceedingly important role in correcting male sexual disorders. It helps in the production of ejaculate, primarily for prostate fluid that makes up much of a man's semen, and in building up testosterone, the male sex hormone, and other body chemicals that help to activate sex hormones.

North American women may be more lacking in pyridoxine than any other nutrient. Certainly ingesting it is a more controllable way of ensuring orgasm than depending on the thoughtfulness or tenderness of your bedmate. In addition, pyridoxine deficiency is one cause of severe symptoms of premenopause and menopause.

The body's sex hormones stimulate such basics of sexuality as vaginal lubrication and penile erection. A short supply of hormones for either partner could have catastrophic effects on your love life. To solve this problem, you must stimulate the endocrine system. Don't do it with drugs or hormone injections, however, but with natural food substances that can rejuvenate the gonads themselves.

Among the finest illustrations of gonadal stimulation is that shown by pyridoxine. This vitamin B-6 plays the most direct role, as a coenzyme, in the synthesis and function of many sex-related hormones. It may be taken as a nutritional supplement or in those foods that contain a high quantity of the nutrient, such as **tuna, lima beans, blackeye peas, navy beans, hazelnuts, pinto beans, bananas, beef, kidneys, chestnuts, spinach, turnip greens, raisins, Brussels sprouts, elderberries, leeks, molasses, Camembert cheese, sweet potatoes, and cauliflower.**

Nutridisiacs for Sexual Slowdowns

Although sexual slowdowns do occur, they are not considered "normal" by sex researchers, most of whom report that sex should actually be more enjoyable as you get older. A woman doesn't even approach her sexual peak until her mid-30s, while men above the mid-40s are able to maintain erections longer to allow for extended periods of coitus.

So why do couples have mid-life crises relating to sex? Investigations by physiologists and nutritionists show that older couples frequently experience a sexually inhibiting decline of hormonal production due, in most instances, to nutritional deficiencies. Simply, the supply of nutridisiacs in their daily food intake is inadequate.

I am convinced, from the research I have done among physicians employing sexual nutrition, that erotic desire and orgasm are the natural expressions of a healthy and vigorous body. When your body is laboring at low-level wellness or subclinical illness, among the first symptoms you experience is a dysfunctioning of your sexuality. Reducing sexual response is nature's way of limiting the human species to the strongest and fittest offspring. Reducing the sexual response of an ill member of the human species is the main way to assure survival of the fittest.

When I interviewed Howard Lutz, M.D., former medical director of the Institute of Preventive Medicine in Washington, D.C., he said: "Anything that promotes good overall health will have a positive effect on a person's sexual desire."

It is unfortunate that many middle-aged individuals erroneously believe that impotence and frigidity are unavoidable consequences of growing older. Instead of learning what is really wrong with their bodies, these sexually-slowed-down people tend to accept a sexual decline as uncorrectable. They do nothing about it, and resign themselves to living without orgasmic sensations. Too bad—and so wrong! While it's true that your body does age and does become more vulnerable to sexual disappointment, this isn't necessarily due to a problem with the sex organs themselves.

The older a person becomes, the more trouble he or she has in absorbing the sexually essential nutrients. Nutridisiacs that you would ordinarily acquire from your daily diet do not get into the blood stream in sufficient quantities. Not enough of a necessary nutrient causes the cells to begin to show evidence of malnutrition by the inadequate performance of the particular organ, gland, tissue, or body part in question. Thus, when older people experience sexual decline, it is usually a sign that there is insufficient nutritional support for the body systems that nourish the sex organs.

Most sexologists assure us that, far from diminishing with age, sexual interest and pleasure actually increase, especially for women. In the September 1981 *Harper's Bazaar*, Armando deMoya, M.D., associate clinical professor of obstetrics and gynecology at Georgetown and George Washington Universities, says: "For those who have always had good sex lives, there may be unexpected bonuses. And for those who have not been fulfilled, these years may bring new discoveries."

"From both a physical and psychological standpoint, the 40s hold the potential for more erotic excitement than ever," adds Anthony Labrum, Ph.D., professor of psychology at the University of Rochester School of Medicine. "However, women sometimes allow the expectation of difficulty to create a self-fulfilling prophecy."

This should not be, of course. The older woman is free from the anxiety of conception and the constant attention drain of young children. She frequently has free time to devote to romance and sexual fulfillment. So, why should sex not be better and more frequent for her? Improper nourishment of one's sexual mechanisms is probably the trouble.

While nutridisiacs cannot change a woman's moral attitude toward sex, the right diet and nutrition level can make her feel better about her body and increase her capacity for enjoyment. A body that is well exercised and at its proper weight can make a woman feel less inhibited and more willing to experiment with new sex techniques. Specific nutridisiacs can be especially helpful, too. For instance, zinc and selenium, both essential minerals, assure a woman of just the right amount of vaginal lubrication during coitus. Also, they preserve the elasticity of vaginal tissues.

For a woman interested in keeping up her sexuality at ages 40, 50, 60, 70, and beyond, being a better lover means maintaining her sexual self by appropriate nutrition. A woman's looks, her vitality and energy are most often cited by men as contributing to her sexiness—far more than any set of sexually arousing techniques. Men also say that women with a healthy capacity to enjoy sex, who can be aroused to orgasm, who are willing to explain their sexual needs, and who are comfortable in a variety of sexual circumstances definitely make for better, more thrilling lovers. The use of nutridisiacs helps a woman acquire these traits.

To overcome sexual slowdown in the middle years, men need to reduce stress levels, get adequate exercise for increasing strength, and supplement their diets with nutridisiacs. Sexual longevity minerals such as zinc, chromium, manganese, magnesium, and selenium should be part of everyone's sexual supplements. Stamina foods such as honeybee pollen, N, N-Dimethylglycine, spirulina, vitamin E, niacin, and ginseng should be taken regularly. Nine times out of ten, the specific cause of a bout of impotence will turn out to be a poor source of nutrition or a lack of particular nutrients in your food.

Nutridisiacs to Restore Erections

Although an occasional loss of erection is not uncommon, the effect can be ego-shattering. Repeated loss will itself make impotence a more permanent part of the man's psyche. It can cause apprehension about future sexual encounters, even if such encounters are with his wife and lover of long standing. In fact, impotence is on the increase in the United States. One in ten is estimated to experience loss of erection with some frequency, and 10 million Americans suffer permanent impotency.

To blame impotence strictly on sexual hang-ups, boredom with the female partner, high stress levels, fatigue, preoccupation with work or outside interests, or other psychological influences is a big mistake. There has been, in my opinion, too much emphasis on the mental aspects of sexual difficulties and not enough on the physical. Emotions certainly play a part in whether or not a man is in the mood for sex, but a wide variety of physical troubles has been overlooked. And once you know what really is causing impotency, the particular physical problem can often be corrected.

Usually, impotence is the result of a lack of an appropriate reflex to a sexual stimulus. Since all reflex actions begin in the brain and nervous system, most sexual problems do start in your head, that's true, but this is a physical disorder and not a mental one. Improving the communication network within the nervous system to attain a better reflex action to sexual stimuli will probably improve the ability to sustain an erect penis, which will, in turn, renew confidence, bring back libido, stoke the fires of sexual energy, and restore feelings of masculine power.

Most of the time, you can improve sexual response and achieve a stronger, firmer, more durable erection by using certain nutridisiacs. In the search for a therapeutic aid to overcome impotence, a recent conference conducted at the White Plains Medical Center in White Plains, New York, on "The Dynamics of Male Sexual Dysfunction" concluded that current treatment provides reversal of erectile difficulty in more than 90 percent of cases.

When the four factors for a normal erection are present, nothing should stop a man from penile expansion. Robert J. Krane, M.D., a urologist on the staff of the medical center at Boston University School of Medicine, lists these four erection factors as "(1) a proper blood supply to the penis, (2) intact nerves that tell the arteries when to open and close, (3) normal erectile tissue capable of filling with blood, and (4) a reasonable emotional milieu." A problem in any one of these four important areas, Dr. Krane points out, can result in erectile difficulty.

In their search for a therapeutic aide for impotence, investigators have checked out blood-vessel bypass operations of obstructed arteries in the genital area; changes in prescribed medications; reduced consumption of alcohol; the use of surgical implants for artificial penis stiffening; controversial hormonal therapy; intravenous injections of a chemical to clean out clogged penis arteries (EDTA chelation therapy); and even a self-contained, remote-controlled electronic device that is surgically inserted in the rectum. Until now, the most popular therapeutic method has been brief, couple-based sex therapy, but some nutritional researchers, including myself, believe there is better treatment available.

At the top of the list of impotence causers is zinc deficiency. Without sufficient zinc, the male body cannot produce enough testosterone, resulting in hormone levels too low to allow for sexual arousal. Furthermore, smoking tobacco and marijuana, drinking alcohol, coffee, and cola beverages, infections, and taking certain medications also deplete zinc reserves and cause erectile difficulties.

Another cause of impotence, especially in men over 45, is low blood sugar. Hypoglycemia indicates that the body's cells cannot get enough sugar from the bloodstream for sufficient fuel. The result is fatigue, irritability, and erectile difficulties. A diet high in protein, moderate in complex carbohydrates (fresh vegetables and whole grains), and the elimination of refined sugar (cake, candy, etc.) can do much to reverse a tendency to impotency. In addition, chromium, the mineral directly responsible for regulating blood sugar, can bring about a sudden and dramatic improvement in your ability to get and sustain a good erection. Chromium helps to keep the blood sugar level normal. Dr. Donald J. Carrow of Tampa, Florida told me: "Adding enough chromium to a man's diet can recharge his sexual batteries."

Chromium may be taken as a sexual supplement in the chelated form, a dosage of 200 mcg of elemental chromium. Or, you can find high concentrations of the mineral in the following foods: **brewer's yeast, beef, calf's liver, whole wheat, including germ and bran, rye, chili, oysters, potatoes, green peppers, eggs, chicken,**

apples, butter, parsnips, cornmeal, lamb, scallops, Swiss cheese, bananas, spinach, carrots, navy beans, shrimp, lettuce, oranges, lobster, blueberries, green beans, cabbage, mushrooms, milk, strawberries, and beer.

Other nutridisiacs recommended by Dr. Carrow are oyster extract, bee pollen, the deodorized garlic extract known as Kyolic, and the wheat germ oil derivative octacosonal, all of which tend to relieve erectile difficulties and revitalize a man's sexual enthusiasm. Furthermore, the fatty acids derived from eating oily fish such as mackerel and blue fish, supplied in the food supplement MaxEPA, help to unblock clogged arteries in the penis, which prevent its spongy tissue from filling with blood. Taking Kyolic and MaxEPA every day causes blood to rush into the penile arteries and the volume of the blood vessels to swell by 200 percent with eight times more blood in the erect penis than in the flaccid one.

Chapter 2

"The Love Pill"

One of the finest readily available food supplements taken internally for enhancing sexual performance is N,N Dimethylglycine (DMG). It had once been designated Vitamin B-15 but, the U.S. Food and Drug Administration ruled that it is not a vitamin at all. It merely appears in nature where other B-complex vitamins are found.

For the past few years, (DMG) has been hailed by nutritionists the world over as a wonder tonic—a revitalizer which, according to *New York* magazine, has served as an energy booster for the likes of Dick Gregory and Muhammad Ali. It's been touted as a fatigue fighter by Dr. Robert Atkins. And now, it's claimed to have an additional benefit: it may help to make a penis thicker, longer, and stronger—and a woman's orgasms wilder.

Frank is a 26-year-old long-distance trucker who has everything going for him. He works for his father, driving a big 18-wheeler, and makes a lot of money. He's good-looking, smart, and possesses a self-assured, open manner that radiates charm. His route takes him regularly to four different cities where girls make themselves available as soon as they know he's hit town. But Frank was concerned with the size of his penis.

No matter how often he had heard that it's not the size of a man's organ but what he does with it that counts, Frank suspected that his penis was not large enough. He had stolen glances of other naked men in locker rooms, shower stalls, and other such places, and judged that what he carried between his legs was smaller than others he had seen.

Consequently, Frank did considerable research on the subject of penis size and growth stimulation, which included visits to physicians who specialize in this sort of thing. And now Frank is no longer unsure of his ability to perform in bed.

Lately, he's had no complaints from a petite blonde he visits in Wilmington, Delaware, or another beauty he frequents in Greenville, South Carolina. Both have noticed an improvement in lovemaking because of the increased size of his penis.

The secret of Frank's new penile enlargement is that he has been supplementing his meals with a particular food substance that makes his penis grow stronger, longer, and fatter. The average flaccid penis is three inches long, but Frank has added a little extra; his erection measures seven inches, one inch larger than average. According to Frank, the added strength, length, and thickness of his swollen member is due entirely to the nutritional supplement he is taking.

Ralph, a 29-year-old merchant seaman, found himself unable to get an erection in the company of a woman during shore leave, although his penis grew stiff when he masturbated in his bunk on board ship. According to noted sex therapists Masters and Johnson, when a man's failure rate to achieve and maintain an erection satisfactory for intercourse approaches 25 percent of attempts, impotence is established. This was Ralph's problem.

Ralph spent time with a behavioral therapist, but that availed no improvement; his trouble was physical—insufficient oxygen circulated to his genitals in the presence of a sexy woman. Because his erotic fantasies were more stimulating to him than sexual reality, any blockage of blood flow into the penis was overcome during his private masturbatory sessions. However, Ralph wanted more.

It was then that he altered his lifestyle; he stopped drinking, smoking, and taking drugs, and under the guidance of a friendly health-food enthusiast—another merchant seaman—Ralph started swallowing vitamins, minerals, other food supplements, and no-junk nutrition. That's when he came upon the nutrient that began giving him fabulous erections. No longer did his penis turn to stone only while fantasizing about exploits with girls that he had met in bars; instead, he began to seek out "nice" women who were often quite willing to explore sex with someone they considered a true "man of the world."

Combining tenderness and passion with a certainty that his penis would respond when required led the seaman to tremendous success and happiness ashore.

The Magic of N,N-Dimethylglycine

N,N-dimethylglycine's biochemical role in the body was originally discovered in 1941 by Philip Handler, Ph.D. The pure food supplement DMG aids in reducing sexual inadequacy caused by subtle and unrecognized malnourishment to the penis. Among other things, DMG provides essential building blocks to the cell and goes into action when foods are transformed into the basic elements your body utilizes for energy or growth; it is a cofactor in your body's metabolism. Known as a nonfuel nutrient, DMG provides a series of biologically active substances required by the energy pool of one's body.

This metabolic cofactor assists hormones, proteins, fats, and vitamins in doing their own job of nutrifying the 60 trillion body cells; and through the same process of nutrition, it frees these cells of toxins. Also important, the movement of molecules stimulated by DMG brings about an increase of the utilization of oxygen held by red blood cells. Since all body cells need oxygen to function, N,N-dimethylglycine is said to significantly enhance one's health—especially sexual health: When more oxygen is required by your excited penis for its expenditure of energy, DMG assists in putting it there.

"DMG, although not a vitamin, should be called the love nutrient, because without it, the love life of many would be empty," says Dr. Lutz. "Women in middle and later years can use DMG to recapture the joys of youth. Men who take it will not only augment their spouse's joy, but their own, as well. Many men who have been inactive sexually find that a period of suitable treatment with taking tablets of DMG allows them to engage in frequent sessions of sexual intercourse—sometimes three or more times daily.

"DMG increases your sexual energy—people lacking stamina do not want anything to do with sex. The penis gets larger, firmer, more lasting with usage, and DMG lets this happen more readily. Although the penis is not actually a

38

muscle, like a muscle, if you don't use it, it seems to atrophy; more use of the organ will make it stronger. If you have a lot of vitality, sexual expression will become easy. There won't be any sexual burnout for you if DMG becomes part of your food supply."

Dr. Lutz says that he uses DMG as a sexual enhancer. He prescribes it to treat sexual inadequacy of various types, including loss of the urge for sexual activity, erectile difficulties, orgasmic dysfunction, and lack of ejaculation.

Taken as a preventive measure against penile problems, N,N-dimethylglycine may work exceedingly well. Since the energy required for the sex act is above and beyond what the body normally needs to carry on life-supporting functions, any lack of endurance could put your love life in jeopardy. Maintenance of body systems in as close to optimum health as possible is the first priority for the body's energy. Only after performing body maintenance will the body spare excess calories to satisfy the sex drive.

Its proponents claim that DMG fights a person's tendency to feel fatigue when the time is ripe for him to engage in sexual activity. The food substance does this by cutting down on waste products, such as lactic acid, which normally build up in the blood when you exercise heavily.

By increasing the amount of oxygen that reaches the penis, N,N-dimethylglycine improves the energy production within your penile cells.

The changing of your penis from the flaccid to the erect state is a natural sexual wonder. It's obvious that the metamorphosis depends not only on healthy blood vessels, but also on a high oxygen level of the blood itself. Cellular efficiency of the penis occurs when plenty of oxygen is present.

Contained naturally in food or as a food supplement, N,N-dimethylglycine is said to improve certain biochemical functions at the cellular level.

According to Jerzy W. Meduski, M.D., Ph.D., a nutritional biochemist in the department of neurology at the University of Southern California School of Medicine, basically, DMG helps the body utilize energy reserves when normal energy sources are too low. Dr. Meduski has been studying dimethylglycine as an important intermediary metabolite since 1976.

Although safe conditions for the use of DMG as a food additive have not yet been established by the Food and Drug Administration, Dr. Meduski determined that the nutrient is exceedingly safe for human consumption; in fact, it is proportionately safer than taking aspirin. DMG is less than half as toxic as table salt, claims Dr. Meduski.

Besides making your penis stronger, longer, and fatter, DMG stimulates the libido, working equally well for men and women. "After a woman has taken DMG," says Dr. Lutz, "even when she has lived in sexual starvation for ten years or more, her response is 'Wow, I didn't know I could feel so wonderful. My sex life is the best ever.'" Orgasms are prolonged and deeper from DMG's ability to transform serotonin (a hormone that constricts the blood vessels) into a substance that does not constrict blood vessels; therefore, blood remains in dilated capillaries and arteries for a longer period during orgasm.

After taking DMG, you may more effectively convert norepinephrine, the hormone for "fight or flight," into epinephrine (adrenaline), which is another major hormone for sexual performance. Without epinephrine, there would be no reaction to even the most exciting sexual stimulus. Epinephrine gets your penis growing when a message from your brain goes out to the various body parts directing them to react to the "reasonable emotional milieu" mentioned earlier by Dr. Krane.

The Endocrinology Laboratory at the Kar'kov Institute Endokrinol, Khim, Formon, in Kar'kov, USSR, under the medical direction of S.V. Maksimove, M.D., has declared that N,N-dimethylglycine stimulates the adrenal glands and regulates adrenal corticoid activity. This means that the nutrient brings about a sexual effect of the two important endocrine glands involved with coitus, the hypophysis and the adrenals.

A final claimed benefit from taking DMG as a food supplement is the improved production of cellular lecithin, required for greater sexuality. Lecithin in the body promotes the secretion of the other various glandular hormones. It assists the passage of substances through the cell walls, producing healthy nerves and efficient mental activity for better sexual response. Raymond Bernard, Ph.D., writes in *The Secret of Rejuvenation* that some European physicians use lecithin to correct sexual weakness, glandular exhaustion, and nerve disorders. Dr. Bernard notes that male reproductive fluid is high in lecithin; therefore, if it is deficient, the sexual powers of virility are simultaneously diminished.

Besides being produced in the body naturally, lecithin is found in l**iver, egg yolks, and raw vegetables.** If you eat insufficient quantities of lecithin-containing foods, popping down a DMG pill may stimulate the formation of natural body lecithin. Of course, before adding lecithin or DMG to your diet—or any other nutritional supplement, for that matter—you should consult your physician or a trained nutritionist.

Indeed, not only the sexually-oriented, but the health-conscious will benefit from the little-known nutrient N,N-dimethylglycine. Properly used, it may give rise to the best erections ever, a tool for heightened sexual pleasure.

N,N-Dimethylglycine comes in tiny white pills of 125 mg each. A pill placed under the tongue will dissolve in about 90 seconds. Take one or two tablets per day in divided doses (morning and evening). DMG is found naturally in **whole grain cereals, corn grits, pumpkin seeds, sunflower and most other seeds, wheat germ and bran, rice bran, liver, yeast, and apricot kernels.**

Chapter 3

Nutridisiacs
For Premenopausal Symptoms

The natural cessation of the menstrual and reproductive cycles in women between the ages of 35 and 60 is known as the time of menopause. Estrogen, the most important female hormone in terms of reproduction and sexuality, stops being produced by the ovaries during and after the menopausal period. Estrogen is responsible for all feminine physical attributes: soft skin, fine scalp hair, limited growth of body hair, thinner and more elongated vocal chords, and preparation for conception by stimulation of the uterus. With the termination of estrogen production, menstruation becomes erratic, and the onset of menopause brings its own set of symptoms.

Symptoms and signs come from the pituitary gland's response to the lowered estrogen levels. It tries, unsuccessfully, to re-stimulate estrogen production. Some women barely notice the body changes, but others are seriously affected by them. The signs of premenopause are flushes, water retention, sudden weight gain, osteoporosis (brittle, frail bones), sleeplessness, and mood swings. The symptoms are hot flashes, depression, uncontrollable crying, and chills.

Hot flashes result from the pituitary's flooding the body with hormones as it attempts to stimulate the ovaries into producing estrogen again. Flashes last from 15 seconds to several hours, and cause sweating, tingling, red patches on skin, and heart palpitations. Another premenopausal burden, one that may trouble your sex life, is vaginal dryness. Estrogen is needed to soften the uterine lining and stimulate menstrual bleeding; it also provides good vaginal lubrication. Poor lubrication can lead to vaginitis (inflammation of the vagina), cystitis (bladder infection), or cervicitis (inflammation of the cervix). It can cause sexual intercourse to become painful and abrasive.

Historically, the most common treatment for easing menopausal symptoms has been synthetic estrogens. It was reasoned that if a woman were going through discomfort due to a sudden loss of estrogen, why not use the hormone to correct the problem? Replacement estrogen therapy (ERT) became commonplace until a higher incidence of uterine and cervical cancer started to show up as a side effect. Women on ERT for seven or more years are 14 times more likely to contract genital cancer than women not using estrogen; women using ERT for one to five years have five and a half times the incidence of cervical or uterine cancer than their non-ERT counterparts.

Saul Gusberg, M.D., a gynecologist at Mount Sinai Hospital in New York City, claims that when estrogen isn't needed for reproduction, the body requires less of it. Eventually, the pituitary and other glands can produce enough estrogen to keep a woman in shape. Consequently, there is no reason to take ERT, especially when the severity of premenopausal symptoms can be directly traced to nutritional deficiencies.

Research among gynecologists working in conjunction with nutritionists points up that the reduction of estrogen depletes a woman's supply of vitamins B-2 (riboflavin), B-6 (pyridoxine), B-12 (cobalamin), folic acid, C (ascorbic acid), and E (tocopherol), as well as the minerals calcium, magnesium, phosphorus, zinc, and chromium. Replacing the lost minerals will reduce the osteoporosis and reduce the potential of acquiring "dowager's hump," the spinal compression resulting in a loss of height, which makes a woman look and feel unattractive. Also, it's necessary to take vitamin B-12 by injection or by eating foods with a high amount of this vitamin, such as **liver, clams, kidneys, oysters, sardines, eggs, trout, brains, salmon, tuna, lamb, sweetbreads, beef, Edam cheese, Brie cheese, Gruyère cheese, blue cheese, haddock, flounder, scallops, cottage cheese, cheddar, mozzarella cheese, halibut, perch, and swordfish.**

The most promising nutridisiacs to combat the direct problems of beginning menopause are ginseng, vitamin E, and oil of evening primrose. Taken in adequate quantities in the time just prior to menopause, these supplements can help most women pass through the period virtually unaffected.

We already know that ginseng stimulates estrogen secretion past the menopausal period. Ginseng also curbs hot flashes and energy loss. The former Chief of the Virus Biology Section at the National Institutes of Health, C.P. Li, M.D., is an exponent of ginseng. Dr. Li said, "The regulatory capability of the body can be made more efficient by ginseng." He went on to explain that during menopause the body is in a state of stress; it is undergoing a temporary endocrine imbalance. Since ginseng contains enzymes and chemicals that naturally stimulate the body to produce more hormones, it helps the premenopausal woman's body to normalize its erratic estrogen production. The dosage of ginseng as a sexual supplement is two 650 mg capsules three times a day.

Vitamin E is an equally excellent natural alternative to estrogen for relieving or eliminating premenopausal symptoms. Warren E. Levin, M.D., medical director of the World Health Medical Group in New York City, said of vitamin E, "Eight years ago I would have prescribed estrogen for premenopausal women to raise their hormonal levels, but I no longer do. A nutritional approach takes longer to produce a measurable effect—about six months—but it can do a better job than anything else."

In addition to daily nutritional supplementation with 400 to 800 international units (IU) of vitamin E (mixed tocopherols are preferable), you can find high concentrations of vitamin E in **wheat germ oil, safflower oil, butter, asparagus, whole rye, carrots, tomatoes, peas, lamb, walnuts, brown rice, salmon, wheat bran and germ, pecans, eggs, and most of the edible seeds.**

Wilfred Shute, M.D., and Evan Shute, M.D., the two prime movers in the use of vitamin E, suggest that prolonged and higher than average doses of this sexual supplement have successfully cured vaginal lesions such as vaginitis, when ERT did not.

Oil of evening primrose is a natural vegetable oil extracted from the evening primrose plant. It is taken as a food supplement in capsule form and is the only source, other than mother's milk, of both the essential fatty acids, linoleic acid and gamma-linoleic acid (GLA), which are the direct precursors for the body's manufacture of prostaglandins (PGE). PGE are hormone-like substances present in a wide variety of tissues and body fluids. A supplemental capsule usually contains 500 mg of evening primrose oil which supplies 40 mg of GLA, 350 mg linoleic acid, and 13 IU of d-alpha tocopheryl (vitamin E).

When evening primrose oil, vitamin E, and vitamin B-6 are taken together by women with painful breast lumps, known as fibrocystic breast disease or cystic mastitis, these women report over and over that the lumps disappear in three or four months. The pain goes away first and the lumps, which may be the size of hardened black olives, steadily get softer until they no longer can be differentiated from normal breast tissue.

Sustaining Sexual Desire as You Get Older

Sexual arousal and desire sometimes go by the wayside as the years go by, but this doesn't have to happen if you use the ultimate nutridisiacs—protomorphogens. The use of sex gland extracts to rejuvenate waning sexual ability is not uncommon among patients of nutrition-oriented sex therapists.

Called live cell therapy, this sex organ rejuvenation technique was first tested and made a scientific reality by the famous Swiss physician Paul Niehans, M.D. (now deceased). Dr. Niehans successfully treated diseased, aging, or non-operative body systems by the introduction of gland extracts from the unborn fetuses of healthy, clinically raised farm animals. Testes concentrates to enhance an aging person's sexuality are being employed today.

Women are now being treated with ovarian and pituitary extracts. And men are responding to concentrates of prostate, testes, and pituitary extracts. This glandular therapy stimulates sexual desire and reverses waning sexuality problems. And there is good scientific logic to why glandular therapy works.

By encouraging the full activity of the sex glands, vital hormone production can be maximized, thereby igniting the body's natural desire and arousal mechanism. The raw glandular extracts, taken as tablets, capsules, and in other supplemental forms, contain a high concentration of nucleic acids, such as RNA and DNA. Plus, the protomorphogens act like the enzymes your cells might ordinarily secrete into the surrounding tissues if they were up to par. They travel to the targeted organ—testicle extract to testicles and ovary extract to ovaries—and the designated organ is stimulated to build new cells and strengthen its own raw glandular concentration.

By themselves, raw glandular extracts are insufficient to prevent premature aging of your sexual apparatus. You still require a nutritious diet and other holistic health recommendations. The protomorphogen properties of raw glandular extracts, however, are effective aids.

Super Sex During Menopause

Though some women may breeze through menopause, the majority experience distressing symptoms. But healthy sex can ease the transition—and even postpone its onset.

Sex not only helps keep the body youthful and vibrant, it also can contribute to a more comfortable menopause. "Most over-40 women will have a less troublesome 'change of life' and even delay its classic symptoms—loss of vaginal lubrication and sensitivity, hot flashes, night sweats, cramping—if they are sexually active," says John Parks Trowbridge, M.D., staff physician at the Northeast Medical Center in Houston, Texas. Though the majority of women pass through menopause without major problems, 75 percent do experience some distress. Along with proper nutrition and a healthful lifestyle sex—either intercourse or masturbation—can provide relief by keeping vaginal tissues toned and moist and releasing endorphins, the body's pleasure chemicals.

The good news is that the 40s can be the most erotic time of your life. The reasons vary widely, but the most basic are hormonal: Estrogen diminishes with age, and the amount of circulating androgens (male hormones)—responsible for fueling the sex drive in both women and men—remains constant. Since estrogen "competes" with and counteracts the effects of androgens, its decline intensifies rather than subdues, desire.

Another physiological plus: The vagina is filled with a cluster of special nerve endings called the venous bed—one focal point of female orgasm - that may become more sensitive with age if a woman continues having sex regularly. And theories suggest that a number of body changes resulting from childbirth can also enhance sexual sensations by the time a woman reaches her 40s.

Some physicians have found that a poor diet, chronic stress and sedentary habits can combine with infrequent sex to intensify emotional disturbances and vaginal atrophy before and during menopause. At the Family Health Center in Indianapolis, IN, David A. Darbo, M.D., prescribes sex and nutrition to reduce menopausal symptoms. He points out the importance of zinc, which affects the oxygen/carbon dioxide exchange in red blood cells. "A zinc deficiency will deprive a woman's tissues of adequate oxygen, which can shortchange her endocrine system and bring on an earlier menopause," he claims. "However, the right mineral level can help stave it off." In addition, the Cowper's gland, which produces a mucus like secretion in women during sexual arousal (as does the prostate gland in men) requires zinc to generate vaginal moisture; a shortage can contribute to internal dryness and painful intercourse.

Master's and Johnson's well-known recommendation for healthy sex—"use it or lose it"—applies especially to menopause, maintains Murray R. Susser, M.D., president of the American Academy of Medical Preventics in Los Angeles. "As with exercise or body building," he says, "sexually conditioning keeps you physiologically fit."

Adds Dr. William J. Faber, medical director of Wisconsin Pain Clinic in Milwaukee: "Keep in mind that consistently 'exercising' a part of the body, like the vagina, increases its blood supply; chronic inactivity, however, can accelerate its aging and deterioration."

Dr. Susser notes that as society has become less inhibited about sex, he has had fewer patients with menopausal complaints, suggesting a link between good sex and an easier menopause. He cites one case in which a woman's long history of calcium loss from premenopausal osteoporosis was arrested by a change in diet, bone-strengthening workouts, and sexual stimulation. He considers the latter a very "efficient" form of exercise: "By generating a natural 'electric current,' vigorous physical activity can help increase calcium formation," he says.

In addition, a steady sex life tones the vaginal muscles that make orgasm possible. In fact, the more the body is accustomed to arousal and orgasmic release, the more readily it responds—so older women who remain sexually active enjoy an erotic advantage.

But perhaps the best reward of sex after 40 is a woman's greater psychological maturity and sensitivity as well as sexual expertise. As women age, they become more relaxed and self-accepting, less worried about living up to others' expectations, observes Lonnie Barbach, Ph.D., a psychologist at the University of California in San Francisco and author of several books on human sexuality, including *For Yourself* and *For Each Other* (both published by Anchor Press/Doubleday). This tolerance enables them to be more adventurous lovers, Dr. Barbach believes. Great sex can take the edge off menopause and make the 40s and beyond your most fulfilling years.

Chapter 4

Beating The Pre-Menstrual Blues

An estimated 80 percent of all women still able to bear children suffer, to one degree or another, from premenstrual syndrome (PMS). Currently the condition has attained medical respectability and popular notoriety. After years of suffering in silence, over a hundred million women in North America now readily admit to experiencing PMS, in many cases a condition that immeasurably disrupts their lives. They and their families will finally be relieved to know that premenstrual symptoms may be biologically reduced or eliminated altogether by the use of certain nutritional supplements, herbal remedies and/or dietary changes.

PMS and its related painful menstruation (dysmenorrhea) are characterized by such symptoms as a heaviness or dull aching in the abdomen, nausea, water retention, constipation, headaches, backaches, breast discomfort, irritability, tension, depression, and lethargy. Frequently the symptoms are relieved by the onset of a women's menstrual period, especially during the heaviest flow. This type of PMS could start at puberty and continue until menopause, often getting worse with each pregnancy.

A New Physiological Basis for PMS

Although doctors might have been taught otherwise, the premenstrual syndrome and congestive dysmenorrhea are real. For centuries menstruating women were accused of malingering when they complained of PMS discomforts. Now we know that the complaint has a physiological basis which accounts for it being relieved by restorative nutrients, soothing herbals and a particular diet.

Hormone-like substances called prostaglandins, which may be released in large amounts in the uterus before menstruation begins, have been cited as the cause of discomfort. Connecticut physicians reporting in *Obstetrics and Gynecology*, the journal of the American College of Obstetrics and Gynecology, advise that a circulating blood factor acts directly on nerve cells or touches off prostaglandin release from various body cells, which in turn causes the PMS reaction.

The doctors proved their discovery by showing that blood plasma drawn from women suffering severe PMS can induce similar distress—abdominal pain, depression and emotional irritability—when the blood plasma is injected back into them at another time. Plasma taken when the donors were not undergoing PMS had no such effect, however. The plasma effect was noted even in women who had undergone a hysterectomy, indicating that one's uterus need not be involved in the reaction.

Nutrients That Reduce PMS

Nutrients introduced that inhibit prostaglandin release and action have brought dramatic relief. Guy E. Abraham, M.D., a former professor of obstetrics, gynecology and endocrinology at the University of California, Los Angeles School of Medicine, The Center for the Health Sciences, has found that vitamin B-6 is extremely effective in minimizing PMS. Dr. Abraham collaborated with Joel Hargrove, M.D. of Columbia, Tennessee, in a six-month-long double blind study with patients suffering from severe PMS. For three out of the six months, their patients received a morning placebo tablet; the other three months they received a daily 500 mg timed-release vitamin B-6 tablet.

"There were 25 patients and the results were that 21 of them had marked improvement when on pyridoxine (vitamin B-6) compared to the placebo," said Dr. Abraham. "Each of the PMS groups of symptoms were substantially reduced. This is a very significant finding when compared to any drug that has been tested."

Earl Mindell, Ph.D., contributing editor and member of *The Vitamin Supplement Journal* advisory panel, in his book, *Shaping Up With Vitamins*, likewise advises the taking of vitamin B-6 for PMS. Dr. Mindell also recommends the daily ingestion of 500 mg of magnesium*; 250 mg of calcium; 300 IU of the dry form of vitamin E, and 1,000 mg of pantothenic acid. To these he adds 500 mg of an herbal, oil of evening primrose, to be swallowed three times a day.

Herbals to Soothe the Symptoms

The herb *dong quai*, two capsules taken three times daily, one-half hour before or after meals beginning a week before menstruation, is suggested by Dr. Mindell as antidoting PMS. He says, "This herb is known as the female ginseng and can improve circulation, regulate liver function, and help remove excess water from the system."

I personally recommend garlic, black cohosh, wild yam, camomile and tansy for eliminating premenstrual symptoms. You can purchase odorless garlic in health food stores as capsules or tablets, or as liquid to be put into your own gelatin capsules. Most of the symptoms of premenstrual tension, according to holistic physicians, are relieved by the daily intake of 810 to 1620 mg of this deodorized garlic, divided into three daily doses.

Black cohosh, native to Canada and the United States, is often called "squaw root" because it was used by the North American Indians to relieve menstrual difficulties. Five grains of the powdered plant stem constitute one dose.

Wild yam made into a decoction (boiling the herb and straining it in the proportion of 50 mg to 100 ml of water) eases PMS.

Camomile is commonly grown in home herb gardens all over the world for its soothing, sedative, and completely harmless tranquilizing effect. It is drunk as a tea to relieve uterine congestions and stimulate the menstrual flow.

Tansy is a robust perennial producing an essential oil that is a valuable agent for various female complaints. Tansy should be taken in small repeated doses as a decoction, powder, tincture, fluid extract, infusion or solid extract on a regular basis before PMS strikes.

Other herbs useful for premenstrual difficulties are red raspberry, cramp bark, blessed thistle, and motherwort. Following is a superb recipe for regulating menstrual flow (to drink during PMS):

PMS Recipe

1/4 ounce true unicorn root
1/4 ounce cramp bark
1 ounce squaw vine herb
1/4 ounce wild yam root

Simmer the mixture for 20 minutes in 1 quart purified water; strain, sweeten with honey to taste, cool, and drink three tablespoons three times daily.

There are herb drinks, teas, tonics, powders, pills, granules, and other mixtures of all kinds for the many sex-related problems.

Treatment of PMS with a Hypoglycemic Diet

Penelope M. Borsarge, R.N., nurse-practitioner in obstetrics and gynecology at the University of Alabama at Birmingham, has successfully treated almost 500 women with premenstrual symptoms using a hypoglycemic diet. She has discovered that PMS patients have difficulty metabolizing simple carbohydrates for one to two weeks before menstruation. In a five-hour glucose tolerance test the women typically develop lower-than-normal blood sugars. Drastic mood swings accompany the nadir in blood sugar, indicating that they are experiencing premenstrual hypoglycemia. PMS episodes typically occur early in the morning, midmorning, mid afternoon, and at bedtime, when a person's blood sugar is usually low.

Mrs. Borsarge has her patients eat six small meals a day rich in protein and complex carbohydrates, with no more than three hours between meals and a bedtime snack of protein and carbohydrate. They are encouraged to eat more **unsweetened fruits, vegetables, whole-grain breads, cereals, low-fat milk, and plain yogurt.** Other suggested foods are **leafy green vegetables, muscle and organ meats, wheat germ and nuts.** Red meat is limited to three meals a week. The diet is high in fiber and low in fat and added sugars.

Patients are urged to avoid caffeine, alcohol and salt. It's recommended that they eat naturally diuretic foods such as **asparagus, cucumbers and watermelon.** Mrs. Borsarge urges PMS women to drink at least six glasses of water a day.

Aerobic exercise is part of PMS therapy. It has a tranquilizing effect that improves the ability to tolerate stress and reduce body fat.

Many women "get through" premenstrual syndrome without paying too much attention to it. But given the fact that some 2000 days of a woman's life are spent menstruating, it's only natural to want no discomfort or anxiety before or during one's monthly period.

Nutrition-oriented physicians suggest honeybee pollen for greater sexual endurance. Bee pollen contains a multitude of natural enzymes, amino acids, minerals, and vitamins—from flowers—that nourish the neurogenital reflex. If you sprinkle bee pollen on your cottage cheese, yogurt, applesauce, or breakfast cereal, your sexual stamina will be increased. Bee pollen comes closest to being nature's perfect food, and an important nutridisiac for its impact on sexual energy.

Lasting sexuality, the stamina for maximum sensual pleasure, the capacity to get the most out of each erotic encounter, and the ability to totally satisfy your lover are attainable through the dynamic combination of body fitness, cellular nourishment, desire, neurological response, and mental programming. These qualities can be maintained and enhanced by taking good care of your body. Sex journal editor Judith Coburn says, "The self-mastery and energy that flow from being in shape make you feel sexier than ever."

*Normally calcium/magnesium supplements are taken in a ratio of twice as much calcium as magnesium; with PMS, twice as much magnesium as calcium is required because a magnesium deficiency causes many of the PMS symptoms.

Chapter 5

The Diet For Fabulous Sex

Our sex drive, responsiveness and stamina is a direct reflection of our good health. We know when we're feeling ghastly that sex is the last thing on our minds. Yet, millions of Americans eat so poorly that their bodies—while not overtly "sick"—are in such a minimal state of health that sex is the first activity to suffer.

Our bodies have evolved slowly with our environment over the past hundred thousand years. But our life style and diet have changed so radically in the last century that our bodies could not possibly adapt. We live in a constant, energy-draining state of stress. The term "homeostasis" describes the way our bodies ideally should be—when all our hormones, body fluids and enzymes exist in a state of perfect harmony. It is in this state that we have the most energy, and we are at our sexual prime. We respond naturally to a sexual stimulus, and we are easily able to satisfy ourselves and our partners.

Anything that throws us out of homeostasis is called a stressor, and we contend with countless stressors every day. Air pollution, anxiety, martinis, illness, trauma, junk food, obesity, extreme heat or cold and toxins are some of the more common stressors which throw our bodies out of whack. Along with our sex lives.

So severe and prominent is this state of minimal health among us that one out of every 10 mature American men is totally impotent. This is an outrageous and frightening number. In fact 50 percent of all American men encounter potency problems more than just occasionally. Hundreds of thousands of women derive little or no pleasure from sex, and often find sex a more painful than pleasurable experience. In a society whose men and women pride themselves on their sexuality and who constantly seek sexual contentment, these numbers are mortifying.

The wonderful irony is that sexual defeat can often be reversed by very simple and basic dietary changes.

Junk Food Impotence

Sugar-laden foods and refined carbohydrates are perhaps the single biggest offenders against an active sex life. In the year 1900, the average American consumed about 11 pounds of sugar a year. Now, he or she consumes more than 125 pounds a year. We get sugar in practically everything: from canned sauces, cured ham and cereal to, of course, ice cream, candy bars and soft drinks. In large quantities, sugar will devastate your sexual drive and potency. While it may momentarily sweeten your taste buds, it can very easily sour your love life.

Refined carbohydrates—white bread, polished rice, noodles, commercial cereals—are just as bad since they break down into simple sugars while still in your mouth. Both sugar and refined carbohydrates rapidly enter your bloodstream where they are converted into glucose, the blood sugar which cells require for energy. Circulating glucose triggers your pancreas to produce insulin, the hormone responsible for bringing glucose into the cells where it's used for metabolic energy.

Because sugar breaks down into energy so quickly, you feel a burst of energy shortly after having a candy bar or soft drink. For this same reason, many athletes "carbo-out" with high-carbohydrate foods just before an athletic event so they have a few minutes of very high energy. But the quick energy often leads to a depressed state right after the sugar is used up.

What happens is that in responding to the huge amount of glucose in the blood, the pancreas produces more insulin than it actually needs. The glucose is rapidly processed, but there's no new supply coming in, and the cells are suddenly left starving for more fuel. When this condition becomes severe, hypoglycemia, or low blood sugar, develops.

Hypoglycemia is one of the most often misdiagnosed, and improperly treated afflictions affecting us today. And it's rising at an alarming rate. Because many of its symptoms are so vague and unspecific, many doctors mistake it for other problems.

Hypoglycemic men do not even awaken with a morning erection, and a complete, rigid erection is nearly impossible for them. Hypoglycemic women have almost no sexual desire at all. Even when they do, they barely have the energy to respond in more than a superficial way. Some misinformed doctors still treat low blood sugar with candy bars. That makes about as much sense as trying to put out a forest fire with gasoline.

What's worse is that left untreated, hypoglycemia often takes a brutal turn toward *hyper*glycemia or too much blood sugar.

Diabetes is only a hop, skip and a jump away, and that's one heck of an unsexy disease. Diabetes itself may not kill you, but it certainly does put a crimp in your life style. Diabetes often brings with it atherosclerosis (hardening of the arteries), which will kill you; kidney damage, which may kill you; and blindness, which can make you *wish* you were dead.

While hypoglycemia and diabetes are the extreme results of sugar-abuse, loss of energy, loss of sex drive, rapid mood changes, depression and potency problems are far more common and likely.

Too much sugar can also directly irritate the sex organs, according to Dr. Henry G. Bieler, author of *Food Is Your Best Medicine*. Sugar-produced toxins often settle in a woman's sex organs while being eliminated through her urinary tract. Sugar makes an excellent medium for bacterial growth, often causing severe inflammation and the formation of putrefactive acids. Simply put, excessive sugar consumption can lead to a not-so-sweet-smelling vagina—a definite sexual turn-off! Intercourse can transfer the irritation to the man's penis, causing subsequent inflammation of the urethra and testicles.

There are numerous ways you can reduce the effects of sugar on your sex life. Chances are you can't completely eliminate refined sugar from your diet. But you should try to reduce intake as much as possible. Cut down on *all* sweets. Try whole-wheat bread instead of white bread. The minerals chromium and manganese have been proven useful in maintaining a proper blood sugar level by increasing insulin's effectiveness so less is needed.

Both these minerals are refined out of most foods, but can be obtained from liver, peas, natural (unprocessed) cereals, whole grains, brewer's yeast (the best natural source) or from chelated supplements available in most health food stores and pharmacies. High-protein foods and supplemental B-vitamins will help repair liver damage caused by too much sugar-produced toxins in the body.

Salt In The Wound

Premature ejaculation is in many cases directly related to excessive salt consumption. Salt is a stimulant. It makes us feel good temporarily by elevating the blood pressure a little and charging up the adrenal glands. But sodium chloride is an ionized element; it has an unstable number of electrons in its molecular structure so it "needs" to latch onto other molecules to stabilize. Sodium chloride is one of the few nutrients which easily diffuses into the cerebro-spinal fluid. Once there, it can disturb the sexual centers of the brain. An imbalance occurs, and loss of sexual control follows. In fact, in addition to affecting sexual performance, excessive salt intake can lead to bouts of temporary violence and insanity.

Salt works hand-in-hand with its counterpart, potassium. For optimal energy levels, a careful balance of nine molecules of potassium to one of sodium should be maintained. Salt abuse is so rampant in this country that the average American has nine sodium molecules to every one of potassium! Salt can aggravate hypertension and cause water retention. Both of these can slow you down sexually. Since salt occurs naturally in many foods, if you can totally eliminate adding extra salt, all the better. Bananas are a wonderful natural source of potassium.

The Great Depleters: Life's Little Pleasures
   Caffeine, alcohol and *cigarettes* are dangerous to your sex drive. The caffeine in coffee, teas, and colas contains cadmium, a toxic trace element that leaches zinc out of your body. Zinc is perhaps the single most important nutrient to an active sex life. Cadmium is a byproduct of the tars in cigarettes, and it floods the smoker's bloodstream as well. Alcohol and caffeine deplete your body of the B-vitamins and vitamin C, all of which are needed to sustain high energy levels while making love. Extra large doses of the B-vitamins and vitamin C will help replace the nutrients you are losing. Reducing your intake of cigarettes, caffeine and alcohol is still by far your best defense.

Preservatives: Embalming Your Libido
   Nitrosamines and other chemical food preservatives will do nothing to preserve your sex life. Beer, cold cuts, smoked fish and meats, and the oils used for cooking french fries and hamburgers are loaded with nitrosamines. In addition to being known carcinogens, nitrosamines are linked to cerebral allergies. Unlike common allergies which cause itching and sneezing, cerebral allergies can affect your mood and dampen your sexual desire.
   Additives in fast foods can lead to impotency, frigidity and a severe loss of libido. Learn how to cook, and be selective in your shopping. The price you pay for convenience may cost you your love life.

Foods That Turn You On

While no one has discovered the ultimate aphrodisiac, there are many foods and nutrients which can *improve* our sex drive and responsiveness. Lots of these are in dangerously short supply in our diets.

Zinc is essential to the manufacturing of testosterone. The average-weight 20 year old male normally has 2.2 grams of zinc in his body, most of which accumulates in his testes. However, as he gets older, he is less capable of absorbing zinc from his foods. In addition, such stressors as smoking, alcohol, coffee, infection and medications will deplete his zinc reserves.

Insufficient zinc results in a low testosterone level—often too low to allow sexual arousal. According to Dr. Carl Pfeiffer, a zinc deficiency can lead to impotency, a greatly reduced sperm count, the improper development of the penis and testes (when lacking in adolescent males prior to puberty) and prostatitis. Zinc is also needed by women to help sustain proper lubrication in the vaginal canal, thus making even vigorous intercourse pleasurable instead of painful.

Dr. Pfeiffer has also discovered large amounts of zinc in the pineal and hippocampus glands in the brain. The pineal gland is directly linked to libido while the hippocampus controls emotions. This leads him to suggest that adequate zinc levels are needed by both men and women for a healthy sex drive.

Oysters are one of the most potent natural sources of zinc, lending some truth to their reputation as an aphrodisiac. **Brewer' yeast, raw eggs, peas, lentils and liver are also good sources for zinc.** Dr. Pfeiffer recommends supplementing 60 mg a day of zinc glutomate to your diet if your normal diet is lacking zinc-rich foods.

Vitamin E plays an important role in carrying oxygen to where it's needed the most. During intercourse, both the clitoris and penis are flooded with blood and need huge amounts of oxygen. Vitamin E helps the blood transport oxygen efficiently and quickly to these organs.

Post menopausal women can help compensate for estrogen loss a lot more effectively and safely with Vitamin E than with Estrogen Replacement Therapy (ERT). Vitamin E can help a woman maintain a very exciting and satisfying sex life through her later years. Women who have had menopause induced prematurely through surgery (hysterectomies or ovary removal) have found it extremely effective in reducing otherwise severe problems cause by sudden estrogen loss.

Vitamin E is found mostly in **unrefined flour products as whole-wheat breads, bran, unprocessed cereals and in nuts, soybeans and wheat germ.** It plays a major role in alleviating vaginitis and preventing prostatitis.

Ginseng users swear by it as a natural sex enhancer. Devotees claim that the only ginseng worth its weight is Korean ginseng, that the American version is a poor runner-up, and the much-hyped Siberian ginseng is really eleuthrococcus, all but useless as a sexual aid. In fact, the Russians feed their own athletes and astronauts only Korean-grown ginseng.

Constant use of ginseng is believed to vastly improve ones virility as well as extend one's overall health and life. One of the ingredients found in ginseng is panquilon, an enzyme that stimulates the endocrine system into producing more hormones. Long term use of the root helps establish a constant supply of hormones needed for sex, energy and stable emotions. Ginseng helps put your body closer to a state of homeostasis. Too, it contains such trace metals as manganese, phosphorus and germanium (used to produce red blood cells) which help provide extra energy.

Users claim that the best source of ginseng is the raw root wrapped in honey to protect it from losing moisture. Simply, eat from the root a few times a day. For those who don't wish to keep a root in their pocket, the next best thing is the thick extract used for making tea. Do not use metal implements with ginseng as they can leach the trace metals right from the extract, thus reducing its potency. Ceramic or wood utensils are best for this purpose.

Protein is a must for energy and for supplying the building blocks needed to make hormones. A complete protein meal is comprised of various combinations of the 22 amino acids. Bee pollen is the single protein food which contains all 22. Other food sources for essential amino acids are **lean meats, fish, poultry, soybeans, lentils, raw eggs yolks, cheese and milk products.**

Strict vegetarians should beware that vegetable proteins lack essential amino acids that our bodies cannot manufacture. These include tryptophan, leucine, isoleucine, threonine, nethernine, methionine, valine and lysine. Protein supplements are necessary for vegetarians. High protein diets create an increased need for potassium and fluids.

Natural sugars, such as honey or fructose, help supply you with energy without the revenge of low blood sugar. Since natural sugars enter the body more slowly than refined sugar they create less of a need for insulin.

Fresh fruits and berries are excellent sources for fructose, and they taste a heck of a lot better than the overly-sweet sugar found in candies.

If You're No Longer Enjoying Sex, The Problem Could Be Your Diet

Your happy sex life is too important to shortchange by neglecting your diet. Knowing which foods can deprive you of an energetic, satisfying love life, and which ones can enhance your sexuality will go a long way in improving your life in general.

Large doses of vitamins, minerals and nutrients alone will not improve your sex life unless the stressful foods and toxins which interfere with it are also reduced. Super-lovers are not supermen or superwomen, they're simply healthy!

The best advice for anyone seeking lasting good sexual experiences is to keep your sexual organs functioning at optimal level through nutrition. Then, all you need is the right partner, time, and place to put your natural machinery into gear. A well-nourished body is, in fact, the ultimate aphrodisiac. How do you acquire a maximally-nourished body? Start with the diet for fabulous sex.

My observation is that a high fat diet (the standard American diet is 45 percent fat) is detrimental to good sex, or satisfactory sex that should be great. Consequently, people who follow the sexual nutrition program my wife, Joan, and I recommend, eat three meals a day, each containing more complex carbohydrates, moderate protein, reduced fat, and almost no refined carbohydrates. My wife and her assistants are helping people achieve longevity and total sexual health through nutrition. Among the tools they use are "The Diet For Fabulous Sex" and "The Seven-Day Fabulous Sex Menu Plan" (or the 14-day, 21-day, and other extended menu plans).

Within a few weeks on this optimal eating plan you should notice an improvement in your sex life, provided your bedmate is following a similar diet.

The foods recommended on the eating program for great sex are: **chicken, turkey, veal, fish, shellfish, liver, lean beef, dried beans and peas, eggs, nuts, natural peanut butter, seeds, all fruit and vegetables (preferably raw or steamed), a limited amount of dried fruit, sourdough and whole-wheat bread, brown rice, whole-wheat pasta, spinach noodles, egg noodles, and cold cereal without sugar or shortening (such as shredded wheat), any hot cereal without sugar or shortening (such as oatmeal), skim milk, cheese made from nonfat milk (such as farmer's cheese or cottage cheese), yogurt, pepper, vinegar, spices other than those prepared with sodium, lemon juice, lime juice, herb teas, filtered water, spring water, unsalted carbonated water, distilled water, pure bottled water, and other purified waters.**

Foods to avoid, or to have only rarely, if you want great sex are **lamb, pork, ham, duck, goose, marbled and fatty meats (such as spareribs and fatty hamburgers), all luncheon meats (such as bologna and salami), all sausages, bacon, frankfurters, kidneys, sweetbreads, hydrogenated nut butters, all fried food, olives, avocados, any baked goods containing sugar and shortening (such as** cake, doughnuts, and commercial mixes), any non-whole grains (such as white rice, white flour breads, or white flour spaghetti), canned milk, fresh whole milk, chocolate milk, cream of all kinds (such as sour, sweet, and whipped), non-dairy creamers, milk chocolate, margarine as a spread, high-fat cheese (such as cream, blue, or Roquefort types), lard, meat fat, salt, pickled products, pudding, sherbet, canned fruit in syrup, gelatin desserts, ice cream, any fried snacks (such as potato chips), shortening snacks (such as pretzels), artificially flavored ices, candy, regular coffee, decaffeinated coffee, regular tea, sugared beverages, colas, artificially sweetened beverages, artificial fruit beverages, and anything at all with additives (if you can avoid them).

Other Aspects of Good Nutrition

Good nutrition must take into account four main principles:

1. Avoid all junk food.
2. Avoid foods to which there is an existing allergy.
3. Eat in such a way as to minimize the response to these allergenic foods to prevent the creation of new allergies.
4. Eat food that is palatable and follow a daily eating pattern which you find most comfortable.

THE SEVEN-DAY
FABULOUS SEX
MENU PLAN

Caffeine, refined sugar, salt, and all fats act as depressants to the sex organs. It is best to limit the consumption of these foods.

Use sunflower oil, safflower oil, or corn oil sparingly for salad dressings and cooking.

The portion size varies with your weight control need.

MONDAY

Breakfast

1 fresh orange
1 poached egg on 1 slice whole-wheat toast
1/2 cup plain-low fat yogurt with nuts and seeds

Lunch

Salad: lettuce, tomato, cucumber, green pepper, and parsley
1 small can of water-packed salmon (drain, remove skin, retain bones)
1 rye roll
1 wedge cantaloupe with 12 grapes

Dinner

1/2 cup vegetable lentil soup
4 ozs. sliced breast of turkey
1/2 cup each steamed carrots and Brussels sprouts
1 small baked potato
1 wedge of fresh pineapple

TUESDAY

Breakfast

1/2 cup each cooked oatmeal, skimmed milk
1 bran muffin
1/2 sliced banana

Lunch

4 ozs. Swiss cheese grilled on pita bread with
4 asparagus spears
Green salad
12 grapes

Dinner

1/2 cup tomato juice cocktail
1/2 cup raw carrots, celery, zucchini, etc.
4 ozs. Shrimp Creole served over 1/2 cup
brown rice
1/2 fresh papaya with lime

WEDNESDAY

Breakfast

1/2 cup plain low-fat yogurt with sliced
mango, sprinkled with chopped nuts, seeds,
wheat germ, and bran flakes
2 rice crackers

Lunch

1/2 grapefruit
4 ozs. broiled trout
1/2 cup each steamed broccoli, carrots
1 whole-wheat roll

Dinner

1/2 cup vegetable bean soup
4 ozs. broiled veal chops
Green salad
1 fresh pear

THURSDAY

Breakfast

1 fresh orange or kiwi
1 egg scrambled in non-stick pan, stuffed
into whole-wheat pita bread

Lunch

1/2 pineapple filled with fresh fruit and
topped with 1/2 cup low-fat cottage cheese
2 whole-rye crackers

Dinner

1/2 cup vegetarian split pea soup
4 ozs. sliced London broil
1/2 cup each steamed cauliflower and beets
Green salad

THE SEVEN DAY FABULOUS SEX MENU PLAN

FRIDAY

Breakfast

1/2 papaya with lime
1/2 cup each cooked whole-wheat cereal,
skim milk
1 slice rye toast spread with 3 ozs. farmer
cheese

Lunch

Chef's salad with turkey and cheese
1 whole-wheat roll
1/2 cup strawberries topped with plain low-
fat yogurt

Dinner

4 ozs. broiled swordfish kabobs with peppers,
onions, and tomatoes served on 1/2 cup
brown rice
Spinach-mushroom salad
1 baked apple topped with raisins, nuts, and
seeds

SATURDAY

Breakfast

1/2 cup low-fat cottage cheese with 1/2 sliced banana and unsweetened crushed pineapple
1 whole-wheat English muffin

Lunch

4 ozs. chicken livers, sautéed in chicken broth, with onions, served on rye toast points
Green salad
1 tangerine

Dinner

1/2 cup barley soup
1-1/4 lb. boiled lobster with lemon wedges
1 small baked sweet potato
1/2 cup steamed green beans
1/2 cup tropical fruit salad topped with sunflower seeds and sesame seeds

SUNDAY

Breakfast

> 1/2 cup stewed prunes with plain low-fat yogurt
> 2-egg omelet with peppers and onions
> 1 whole-wheat bagel

Lunch

> 1/2 cup multi-bean soup (black, navy, pinto, lima, red, etc.)
> Green salad with flaked tuna and rye croutons
> 1/2 grapefruit

Dinner

> 4 ozs. Chicken Teriyaki (marinated in orange juice, soy sauce, garlic and ginger)
> 1/2 cup each stir fried assorted fresh vegetables
> Brown rice
> 1 wedge honeydew melon filled with fresh cherries

Chapter 6

Fabulous Sex For 120 Years

*In the sacred valley of Vilcabamba, high in
the Andes Mountains of Ecuador, the people
often live to 120 years, remaining strong,
healthy, libidinous, and actively working
until the last months of life. They possess
longevity and sexual secrets which I am
revealing now, long after my visit to their
mountain home. What you are about to read
is documented in the scientific literature and
comprises my first hand experience.*

In 1981, the government of Ecuador was
seeking a means of exchanging its product and
services internationally in order to acquire imports
and attract foreign investment. After months of
evaluation the bureaucrats settled on mineral
deposits as the chief means of bringing in foreign
exchange.

Ecuador's mountainous terrain, is the source
of an enormous amount of minerals which are
exceedingly difficult to extract.   Until then,
petroleum, sulfur, and gold were the only important
commercial exports.

During mineral explorations, some of the nation's government officials discovered that the world was intrigued with another of Ecuador's natural wonders—one of the country's many mixed Spanish/Indian tribes tucked away in a remote tropical paradise near the southern border which legend has designated as the biblical "Garden of Eden." It was snuggled in a valley at 4,000 feet altitude and surrounded by the Andes range of mountains that rise above 14,000 feet. Here lies the village of Vilcabamba.

Los Viejos (the Old Ones) of Vilcabamba

One of the amazing facts about this village, which I discovered when becoming part of a scientific expedition and visiting there in November 1981 as the party's assigned medical journalist, was that out of a population of 814, approximately 15 percent of the people were over 90 years old. At least 14 of them were centenarians, and one of these Vilcabambans was the oldest living person in the Western Hemisphere. Not only that, at age 132 Jose Maria Roa was married to his third wife, a young chick of 67 named Mariana, and they routinely enjoyed sexual intercourse a minimum of twice weekly. She had given birth to the elderly fellow's 23rd child just 15 years before. In fact, she was still menstruating.

Having sex serves a dual purpose for the century-old villager and his matriarchal wife. Senor Roa said not only does it help him fulfill "God's will", but he and his partner reach orgasm and sleep better at night.

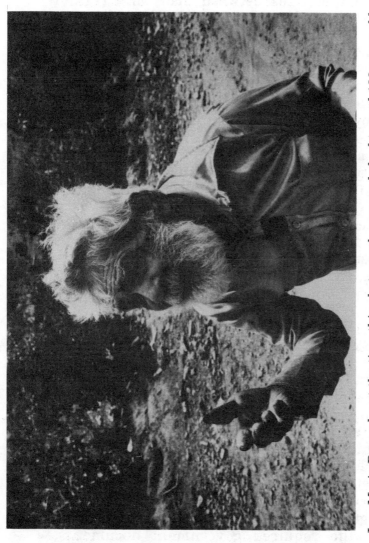

Jose Maria Roa, who at the time this photograph was made had turned 132 years old. He still worked in the fields picking snap beans, and his sexual life remained active. In fact, when his sperm was tested at 119 years of age, Jose Maria Roa still had viable spermatozoa and could impregnate a woman.

Neither Mariana or Jose Maria Roa thought it unusual that sex between them on a regular basis was standard procedure. That's because among all of the elderly residents, including those others ages 120, 109, 105, 102, active participation in sexual intimacy was as essential to living as eating, drinking, sleeping, and excretion. I was able to learn this in a kind of town hall gathering called by the village leaders eight days after my party of scientists arrived. Ours was a government-sponsored visit for medical, sexual, longevity, and other scientific investigations, and we had the trust of Los Viejos (translated from the Spanish, it means "The Old Ones"). They had benevolent feelings for their Ministry of Health who treated the villagers like national treasures and sent them sustenance in the form of clothing, farm animals, and tools on a regular basis.

My Expedition to the Long-Lived Villagers of Vilcabamba

So, officially under Ecuador's protection, my wife who came along as an assisting journalist, myself, and an accompanying group consisting of an affable Spanish interpreter, a medical gerontologist from South Africa, a Scandinavian geologist, a British sexologist, a nutritionist, an anthropologist from Mexico, a couple of Ecuadorian soldier guides who doubled as security guards (they carried the required government documents, machetes and guns), all engaged in this expedition over the lower slopes of the Andes Mountains and through dense jungle. While the jungle was torrid, the higher crests were snow clad. Still where we were heading, an inter-Andean basin, the climate was to prove comfortable and spring-like with little variation throughout the whole year.

In Vilcabamba, there are two seasons only, the rainy, lasting from December to May, and the dry, lasting from June to November. More children are born in Vilcabamba nine months following the rainy season because sometimes the tropical rains are so heavy it's difficult for even these hearty villagers to get out into the fields for working. So they stay home in their snug adobe huts and make love.

We arrived when the dry season was ending and the road dust made automobile travel absolutely hazardous. The driver found it impossible to see even 20 feet in front of a vehicle. So we drove very slowly with lights on in the daytime even though we were just three degrees from the equator and the sun was bright orange and hot.

Our specific purposes for being there was to learn from the Vilcabambans the secrets of their long sexual lives. I wrote articles for publication in a half-a-dozen health-type magazines. One of my articles appeared in <u>The Globe</u> and elicited thousands of queries to the tabloid which subsequently were forwarded to Ecuador. Another of my pieces appeared in <u>Lion's International Magazine</u>, since I witnessed and photographed the induction (I was a Lion's Club member at the time) of that oldest living human in the Western Hemisphere.

What better place to make our investigations about the secrets of prolonged sexuality and long life than a location on earth where the population habitually lives the full complement of mankind's years—where they get maximum usage from the human genetic code. Here we were about to record interviews with a people known as <u>Los Viejos</u>. I did interview them and did take about 600 photographs during our expedition.

Moreover, Garry F. Gordon, M.D., now practicing medicine in North Highlands, California, but who was then medical director of the Hayward, California diagnostic laboratory, MineraLab, Inc., learning of Joan's and my forthcoming excursion, volunteered to perform soil, water, "Panella" and hair mineral analyses on specimens with which I would return and ship to him. MineraLab did perform those analyses, and the knowledge gleaned, which I fully documented and published in <u>Secrets of Long Life</u>, brought another advancement for nutritional medicine.

In summary, we learned that human tissues really do become what is ingested by a person in the form of food and drink, especially if high-mineral-content, pristine drinking water is part of that ingestion. Also, we uncovered that even if one sits on a mountain of aluminum, which <u>Los Viejos</u> do have as part of their ecology, an individual state of homeostasis holds off degenerative diseases of all types. For example, Alzheimer's disease, diabetes, atherosclerosis, cancer, arthritis, cataracts, impotence, and nearly all other pathological degenerations are unknown among the long lived people of Vilcabamba.

Even women 100 years old and beyond regularly experience orgasms. Indeed, the sexologist discovered that the ability to orgasm for the elderly men and women remain with them even when they are ill. A 96-year-old Vilcabamban man may be lying in bed with two broken legs from having fallen from his horse, but while there recuperating in the village's three-room hospital or in his hut high on a hillside he will get an erection and be looking for female companionship.

Los Viejos die eventually, of course, but the causes of their deaths are either iatrogenic—caused by a medical doctor—(e.g. administering antibiotics) or accidents (e.g. plunging down chasms) or from their bodies simply wearing out after 12 decades or more.

We Interview 132 Year-Old Jose Maria Roa

Joan and I arrived at our destination after an 11 hour jet flight to Guayaquil, Ecuador. Then we experienced another more hair-raising 45-minute flight in an Apache single-propeller, light aircraft at 8,000 feet which passed between mountain peaks rising double that altitude above us. Next we took a bumpy drive in the back of a rickety open truck for a couple of hours after leaving the airstrip near Loja (caged chickens were our truck companions). Over Joan's protests each of us sat astride burros as we ascended and descended steep mountain passes. Then we were forced to trudge through jungle growth hacking our way with machetes to finally arrive at Vilcabamba.

We found Jose Maria Roa in his field 2,000 feet up the mountainside. It was approximately 8,000 feet above sea level where the air is thinner but pure and brisk. An energetic man, he was short—just over five feet tall—white-haired, and full of humor and good will. His spirit was high, and he attacked his bean-picking with zeal. The climb from his cabin, although I considered myself in excellent physical condition, was exhausting. We are hikers, but it took my wife and me almost two

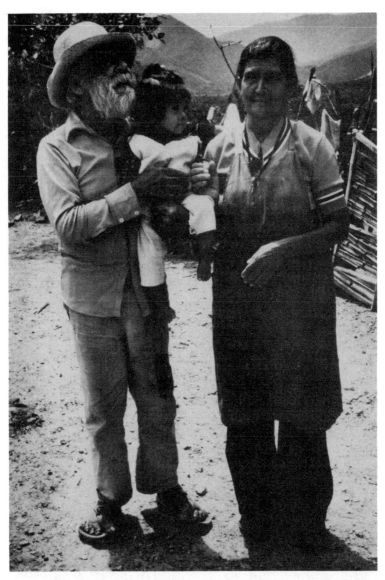

Jose Maria Roa stands next to his third wife, a young chick who is 67 years old. She is still menstruating. Most Vilcabamban women continue to menstruate until well past 70 years of age. Jose Maria Roa is holding one of his dozens of great, great, great, grandchildren.

hours to travel the distance. Jose Maria Roa made this ascent every day, and then put in eight hours of vigorous labor pulling out stumps, chopping wood, hand tilling his corn, string beans, sugarcane, coffee beans, and fruit trees, and doing the myriad other tasks that made a Vilcabamban farmer successful. It was hard work which Roa had been doing for more than 120 years.

On that November day of our visit Jose Maria Roa was 132 years old, as I mentioned married for the third time to a woman who was then 67, and who gave birth to Roa's youngest son 15 years before. The Ecuadorian government verified these facts and the Spanish interpreter who was supplied to us by the Ministry of Health, presented us with Roa's birth certificate that indicates he was born in 1850. Also, we saw that his name was carved into the foundation stone of the church sitting in the center of Vilcabamba. Roa helped erect that structure in 1866. He and the other old ones of Vilcabamba were valued like Spanish doubloons or precious gems.

Los Viejos stayed youthful, sexual, and active until the moment of death. Simply put, they died young at a very old age. The centenarians achieved this hearty longevity by living an inordinately healthy lifestyle, compared to populations in industrialized countries. Statistics. show there is one person over 100 years or age for every 1.7 million Americans. In Vilcabamba, it is one in 68.

Why Los Viejos Live so Long and Stay so Sexy

These people lived long and remained sexually active for several reasons. They exercised vigorously every day, as this was the only way to

89

earn a living as farmers. Their work had them bending repeatedly and using their abdominal muscles in a series of contractions and relaxations. Such abdominal activity pumps the arterial blood flow and causes a good nutrition to surge through the pudendal artery into the genitals. Alternate in and out contraction of the abdominals with constant flexion of the pudendal arterial walls does not allow for blockage of blood flow to the penis or clitoris. Consequently, when sexual excitement occurs for one of the old ones, the sex organ of intimacy is ready to react. Their libidos stay high and their organs continue to be sensitive—all from nutrition furnished by their excellent blood flow.

They didn't own any motorized equipment, and all of their tending of the soil had to be accomplished with hand tools with the subsequent muscular contraction and relaxation involved. In the Andes, there is no level land for planting except for what might be scratched out of the jungle.

In the United States and other Western countries there is no natural environment or other arrangement that is quite like that in Vilcabamba. But there are devices which do tend to stimulate blood flow through the pudendal artery and into the male or female genitals. A particular organization that has dedicated itself to improving the blood flow for generally unhealthy Americans, especially those with cardiovascular disease, has developed a device that improves blood flow through the abdominal aorta and other arteries in the lower quadrants of the body. The Association for Cardiovascular Therapies, Inc. has created a small belt-like device that wraps around the abdomen with a spring mechanism that allows you to flex and contract your abdominal muscles in a periodic series of movements. This movement forces firm and

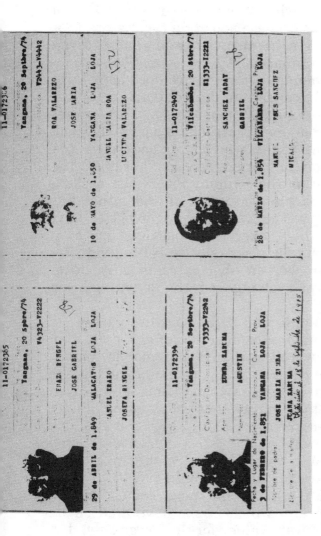

Shown are the birth certificates of four Los Viejos with Jose Maria Roa's depicted in the upper right. He was born the 10th of May 1850, and his name is inscribed in the cornerstone of the village church, erected in 1866, as one of the builders.

healthy pressure on the walls of the pudendal artery so as to push arterial blood downward to the penis or clitoris. These sensitive organs are then well nourished with nutrition and ready to rise upon sexual stimulation.

The pudendal artery device does something else. It's use causes active contraction of the abdominals and makes them strong. Flab around the stomach area disappears, and a person develops a flat abdomen. Excess weight gain goes away, too. The Association for Cardiovascular Therapies, Inc. calls its invention the "Tummy Sizer" just because it accomplishes this reduction of abdominal flab and flattening of the waist. It might better have been named the "Sexersizer" because use of it achieves orgasm for a sexually active individual— especially for women—better than any other mechanism ever evolving from the inventive brain of man.

The people of the sacred valley of Vilcabamba have absolutely no air pollution, because there were less than 20 automobiles known to exist among the entire population during the time of our visit. We saw that burros and oxen were the beasts of burden, but people also did a lot of the burden-carrying.

There were no industrial factories of any kind unless one would consider the making of "panella" sugar cane candy an industry.

They ate almost no meat except for an occasional chicken which might have died on its own. Chickens were valued for their eggs only. Los Viejos' food supply came only from fresh fruits and vegetables which they raised or picked wild. It was with delight that Joan and I discovered that we needed but to reach out our hands to gather the berries, mangos, papayas, grapes, lemons, oranges, apples, pineapple, crab apples, and other wild-growing assortments readily available. Indeed, nobody starved in Vilcabamba, for potatoes, carrots, plantains, breadfruit, cucumbers, zucchini, citrus, little apple-bananas, regular big bananas, coconuts, and a great deal of other edible plant life grew wild everywhere. It thrived without cultivation, except for a few items that farmers wanted to bring to the table. There were avocados, legumes, rice, all of the other grains, tomatoes, cabbage, eggplant, squash, and much more. Canned foods were never used, and we wondered how the single grocery store in town continued to stay in business.

There was no refrigeration. Food had to be eaten fresh and usually raw. <u>Los Viejos</u> did smoke tobacco but it was cured pure with no additives and wasn't wrapped in paper as are cigarettes. Rather, they smoked small leaf-wrapped cigars. Furthermore, they drank a fiery grain alcohol called <u>Aquadiente</u> that burned the lips, the tongue, the palate, the throat and the stomach all the way down one's gullet, and the burning remained long past the liquor's last swallow. It probably acted as a detoxifier to kill any unfriendly microorganisms coming in contact with the stuff.

Analysis of Vilcabamban Soil, Water, "Panella" and Hair Tissues

According to Dr. Garry Gordon's MineraLab analysis of the samples my wife and I brought back to the United States at the end of our two-week expedition, the old ones consumed a combination of multiple minerals in their food and water. Unlike the body mineral content of Western industrialized people, the Vilcabambans showed perfect ratios of certain essential minerals in their samples. The contents of soil, water, "panella" and hair exactly matched each other in concentration of minerals. The Vilcabambans were undoubtedly comprised of exactly what they ate and drank.

Dr. Gordon, who supervised the analysis, said, "As we look at the total picture of these elderly people, the hair tests show that they are not victimized by the same degenerative diseases such as cancer, diabetes, heart disease, and arteriosclerosis, so prevalent in our own citizens . . . The minerals they drink in their water supply seem to be their natural protection."

In Vilcabamba, the water gathers in mountaintop lakes at 14,000 feet and rushes down rocky precipices. Collected in artesian wells lying just under the ground at 4,000 feet in the sacred valley, this water has the perfect balance of minerals apparently needed for longevity—selenium, chromium, zinc, manganese, potassium, calcium, magnesium, and others.

Each of these minerals played a specific role in keeping the old ones productive, in sound condition, and youthful. Selenium, for example, may have been the major influence in the continued sexuality and incredible long lives of three women that we met. Felicia Herrera was age 104; Margarita Aliaga was 103; and Anita Guaman was the youngster at 100. Each woman had the ideal quantity of selenium showing in her hair following its analysis by Dr. Gordon. Joan was the secretary in this research and kept careful recordings of our soil, water, "panella" and hair collections. All of the women were active homemakers and assisted their children in the fields. With a prodigious average of twelve children each, we can safely assume that they led and were still leading active sex lives.

Furthermore, through our Spanish interpreter, they all reported not reaching menopause until after age 70!

Selenium was also likely to have been the main mineral that had kept Los Viejos from suffering from cancer of any kind. In fact, when we described the symptoms of breast cancer to the three women just described, they thought the whole crowd of us were joking—even the anthropologist who was a very serious fellow. Breast cancer is just unknown in the sacred valley. And a description of Alzheimer's disease was believed by all of Los Viejos to be another joke, even with assurances coming from our official translator who worked for Ecuador's Ministry of Health.

The not-so-wrinkled appearance of hard-working, 102-year-old Eduardo Gonzales may result from adequate selenium. Because selenium is an antioxidant, it tends to preserve elasticity of skin tissues, which probably accounts for the centenarian having somewhat youthful look to his face despite his advanced age. The amount of wrinkles Senor Gonzales displayed appeared about the same as an American man who was 72 years old.

Now Eduardo Gonzales has an interesting sex history. He does not farm but rather buys his produce with money that he earns from pushing a wheelbarrow or splitting big stones into little ones with a pickax. He is part of the road-building crew which makes up the public works department of the southern district of these Andes Mountains. It happens that Eduardo Gonzales admits to thinking of making love with different women while he pours cement or carries bags of sand for the road work. He is unmarried but does own a good hut for sleeping and entertaining visitors, he says. His greatest pleasures are being able to provide for his own provisions and asking sexual favors of different women in the town. Every night he invites in a different woman to share his food and then his bed. Even with the back-breaking labor he performs all day, 102-year-old Eduardo Gonzales is never too tired for lovemaking.

More Sexuality Among the Old Ones

Besides selenium, zinc is another mineral which may have helped to preserve the youthful faces of the Vilcabambans. It, too, is involved in keeping the skin tissues healthy and elastic. However, more importantly, zinc was probably why the inhabitants of the hills surrounding the sacred valley maintained their male potency, female climatic, and enthusiasm for sex for so long.

One case in point was Damon Lanche, then age 109. A very active Vilcabamban who worked every day in his corn fields, climbing 2,600 feet to get to them, Damon described himself as still sexually potent. After his wife died five years before, he claimed to habitually pay visits to the town's many women for purposes of sexual relief. His focus. like Eduardo Gonzales, was spent all day on what he would do with the woman he would have for the evening.

Let me clarify that during our visit we learned that prostitution was not considered dishonorable or any sort of crime in Vilcabamba, rather, it was accepted as a necessary service rendered in exchange for money. In that part of Ecuador, it was a form of Social Security for unmarried women—widows, spinsters, divorcees. Age was no factor in their rendering such services and the local society of husbands and wives just accepted it as the natural way of living. Women as old as 90 years were accepted as town women and fully employed as long as they had strength to deliver services.

We climbed to the cabin of Manuel and Eleanora Ramon who resided on an outcropping of rock at 6,000 feet. Having brought a supply of Western goodies (baddies) unknown to the taste buds of the Ramons, our party remained for lunch and were treated very hospitably by them. In fact, all of us shared intimacies in order to get Senor and Senora to talk about their everyday activities of working, church attending, and recreational pursuits.

Strictly for purposes of the anthropological record and to help the Ministry of Health in Quito keep a census of its citizens, 118-year-old Manuel Ramon stated openly to the sexologist without boasting, and 105-year-old Eleanora concurred, that they enjoyed sexual intercourse together a minimum of twice a week. It was the usual pattern as with all of the Vilcabambans no matter what their ages. Sexual intimacy at least twice in seven days was standard procedure for these very natural people.

"You see," Manuel explained, "when the sun goes down, there is nothing else to do." They have no electric light for reading and most of the mountain people rise with the first light of dawn and go to bed as soon as the sun sets.

"For a man who is well into his second 100 years of life", said the cheery interpreter as Manuel listened, "you seem to enjoy living to the fullest—more than most."

"No, not so! I don't behave with my woman any differently from other married neighbors whom

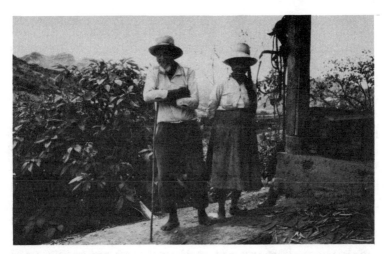

Senor Manual Ramon, age 118, and his 105-year-old wife, Senora Eleanora Ramon standing outside their adobe brick home atop a mountain outcropping at 6,000 feet elevation.

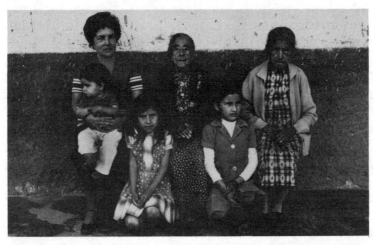

The unusual gathering of four out of five female generations: In the center is 112-year-old Simone Juarez; to her left is her daughter, Philhamena, who looks older than the mother; to Simone's right is her granddaughter Anna; the great granddaughter, Juanita, is not present because during the day she works in the fields potato-farming; Juanita's three children are shown, and they are Simone's great, great grandchildren.

God has bound together," said Manuel Ramon. "Sex relations with one's woman is a need the same as are eating, breathing, and sleeping." It was a refrain we had heard before. Such a philosophy is ingrained in the people who are highly religious and earthfully accepting of their sexuality.

The Vilcabambans are Ecuadorian Indians who practice Roman Catholicism. They attend church services faithfully every Sunday. Besides occasional livestock auctions conducted in the village, church going is their chief form of diversion.

Conclusions About Los Viejos

While each of the multiple minerals present in equal concentrations in the tissues, drinking water, soil, and "panella" of the Vilcabamba population has a specific life-giving and youth-enhancing function, our investigations kept coming back to the amazing fact that Los Viejos are free of the diseases that usually cut short the life spans of Westerners.

Heart disease is unknown in this population. The reason, we believe, is due to the overall synergistic workings of the minerals in the Vilcabamban drinking water. Somebody ought to bottle it and sell the pristine liquid as a health tonic. Sufficient amounts of magnesium is able to help break up the arterial plaque that causes atherosclerosis. We know that it also works better as a coronary spasm blocker than even calcium channel blocking agents. Chromium in the water along with manganese, calcium, and potassium are there together maintaining regular heartbeat.

In addition to the lack of heart problems, the participants in my expedition also found the old ones to be essentially free of blood sugar ailments like diabetes and hypoglycemia, cancer, and arthritis.

Significantly, the old ones never heard of senility. These Vilcabambans remember and have alert minds until the day they die.

As for lack of climax for a Vilcabamban woman or impotence for any of the elderly men, it just does not exist. Everyone enjoys their sexual activities to the fullest, since it is the most natural experience given to them by God. Visiting the Los Viejos of Vilcabamba was an inspiration.

In the next chapter you are provided with listings of herbs and foods which offer nutridisiacs for fabulous sex. These are the secret tools applied to the long-lived people of Vilcabamba who enjoy sexual intimacy until the day they die. Actually, these are not secrets at all because the old ones readily shared their information with members of my scientific expedition. Use the information, enjoy restoration of a potentially lost sexuality, and live a long and full life like Los Viejos.

Alert, active and involved, Jose Maria Roa, Manuel Ramon, Eduardo Gonzales, Damon Lanche, and all the other centenarians, should serve as reminders to everyone that life can be lived healthily and happily with the benefits of good nutrition and exercise, and importantly, an environment that focuses on every individual's personal well being. It's the secret of longevity with prolonged sexuality.

Chapter 7

Herbs And Foods

The Vilcabambans live off the land. They have no health food stores available to give them nutrients in pills, powders, capsules, tablets, spantials, drops, or other forms of nutritional supplements to heighten sexuality. Their nutridisiacs come from the foods they eat and the herbs they administer. As a result, their naturalness and dependency on what grows in the land patches they cultivate or from what is found growing wild in the jungle becomes the nonscientific or unsophisticated way that they live. It's simple and their method works, for they are the longest living and most sexual human beings on earth.

How do they accomplish this record of success in living? They ingest wholesome herbs and foods that have their bodies and minds functioning homeostatically. They are holistic consumers of nutritional components.

In this chapter you will be offered many listings of the nutritional values of foods that are available in Western societies which make up North America, Europe, Australia, and large parts of Asia and Africa. My recommendation is that you carry these listings to the supermarket, grocery, and other points of food selection. Choose your edible products by estimating the nutridisiac value of the foods offered for sale. It means making intelligent decisions about what you are bringing home. But remember, what you put in your mouth does become you. Eat garbage and you become garbage. Consume the best and you become the best.

Herbs Used by <u>Los</u> <u>Viejos</u> for Better Sex

There are at least 800,000 species of plants on earth, only a fraction of which have been studied for medicinal qualities. About 40,000 are now under study to determine their nutritional value; probable 20 percent of these can be used to promote better health. The following list of herbs and combinations of herbs is necessarily limited because we want to focus on plants that have sex-related benefits. The herbs listed on the following pages are helpful in treating sexual problems. More information about each individual herb listed can be found in books on herbology.

Herbs to Cure Impotence and Increase Sexual Power

Arrach
Burr gockeroo
Damiana
Betal
Camphor
Echinacea
False unicorn
Garden sage
Guarana
Jamaica ginger
Murira-puama
Night-blooming cereus
Nux vomica

Quaker button
Summer savory
Sundew
Vanilla pods
Virginia snake root
Yohimbe
True unicorn
Black cohosh
Ginseng
Carline thistle
Matico
Coca
Saw palmetto berries

Herbs to Normalize Menstrual Function

Acacia
Aloe
American centaury
American pennyroyal
Ammeniacum
Arbor vitae
Asafetida
Balm
Bayberry
Beet
Birthwort
Bistort
Bittersweet
Black cohosh
Black hellebore

Black horehound
Blessed thistle
Blood root herb
Beneset
Brooklime
Buckbean
Button snakeroot
Cajuput oil
Calamint
Catnip
Cedar berries
Columbine
Comfrey
Contrayerva
Cotton root

Crawley root
Cubebs
Dandelion
Devil's bit
Dyer's madder
Elecampane
European ground pine
European pennyroyal
Evening primrose
False unicorn
Fenugreek
Fever root
Figwort
Fringetree
Garden sage
Garlic
Gentian
German camomile
Goldenrod
Golden seal
Ground pine
Guaiac
Hemlock spruce
Horehound
Jacob's ladder
Jamaica dogwood
Jerubeba
Jerusalem oak
Lavender cotton
Lemon
Life root
Linden
Lovage
Lungwort
Mandrake
Manganita
American angelica

Bamboo juice
Arrach
Bethroot
Bitter root
Masterwort
Black haw
Mistletoe
Black mustard
Myrrh
Blue cohosh
Peach
Buchu
Peruvian rhatany
Barnet
Plantain
Camomile
Pulsatilla
Carrot
Red raspberry
Celandine
Rue
Cornflower
Sanicle
Cramp bark
Savin
Culver's root
Shepherd's purse
Double tansy
Sneezewort
European angelica
Southernwood
Fennel
St. John's wort
Feverfew
Stramonium
Galbanum
Summer savory

Gelsemium
Sweet marjoram
Ginger
Tamarack
Gravel root
Tansy
Guarana
Turkey corn
Horsemint
Vervain
Jamaica ginger
Wake robin
Juniper berry
White bryony
Lemon thyme
Wild carrot
Lobella
Wild marjoram
Magnolia
Wintergreen
Marigold
Wood sage
Mayweed
Yellow flag
Motherwort
Santonica
Oregon grape
Scabiosa
Peppermint
Slippery elm
Pilewort
Solomon's seal
Pleurisy root
Spruce
Ragwort
Stinging nettle
Red sage

Sumach berries
Saffron
Sweet cicely
Meadow lily
Sweet-scented
    goldenrod
Mugwort
Tanacentum
    balsamita
Parsley seeds
Thyme
Peruvian bark
Uva ursi
Pitcher plant
Valerian
Prickly ash
Virginia snakeroot
Red cedar berries
Watercress
Rosemary
White pond lily
Safflower
Wild columbine
Sassafras rootbark
Wild mint
Senega
Witch hazel
Smartweed
Wormwood
Sorrel
White ash
Squaw vine
White poplar
Storax
Wild indigo
Sumbul
Wild yam

Sweet gale
Wood betony

True unicorn
Yarrow

Herbs to Help Prevent Abortion

Cramp bark
Lobelia

Witch hazel
Red raspberry

Herbs that Slow Down Sexual Function and Desire

American black willow
Black willow
Celery
Cocoa
Hops
Life everlasting

Scullcap
White pond lily
Camphor
Oregon grape
Garden sage

Herbs to Stimulate Uterine Contractions and Expedite Birth

American angelica
Bethroot
Birthwort
Black cohosh
Blue cohosh
Cedar berries
Cinnamon bark
Cinnamon oil
Cotton
Cotton root
Cramp bark
Crawley root

Honeysuckle
Horehound
Lobelia
Red raspberry
Rue
Spikenard
Squaw vine
Sweet gale
Shepard's purse
St. John's wort
Uva ursi

Herbs to Relieve Symptoms of Veneral Diseases

America senna
Barberry
Bitterroot
Bittersweet
Black walnut
Black willow
Bloodroot
Blue flat
Boldo
Boxwood
Burr gockeroo
Button snake root
Chaparral
Cleavers
Copaiba
Corn silk
Cubebs
Culver's root
Echinacea
Elder bark, leaves & berries
European birch
Fringetree bark
Galla
Golden seal
Hardhack
Hydrangea
Indian sarsaparilla
Ivy
Kavakava
Krameria root
Life everlasting
Manaca
Manganita

Marshmallow
Matico
Mosereon
Mullein oil
Oregon grape
Pareira
Parsley
Peruvian rhatany
Pipsissiwa
Poke root
Prickly ash
Red clover
Red raspberry
Rock rose
Sandalwood
Stillingia
Storax
Soapwort
Spikenard
Sarsaparilla
Sassafras rootbark
Tag alder
Thyme oil
Tragacanth
Turkey corn
Twin leaf
Uva ursi
White pond lily
White poplar
Yellow dock
Yellow parilla
Bayberry
Marhs rosemary

Black catechu
Mountain laurel
Bladderwrack
Pansy
Blue violet
Peruvian balsam
Burdock
Plantain
Caroba
Quince
Condurango
Red root
Cranesbill
Sanicle

Devil's bit
Shavegrass
Frostwort
Spruce
Guaiac
Sumach, berries & leaves
Hyssop
Tormentil
Juniper berry
Turpentine
Lily-of-the-valley
White pine bark
Mandrake
Wild sarsaparilla

Food That Contains Vitamins for Better Sex

The quantity of each item on the following lists has been standardized to 100 grams, which provides a more appropriate comparison between relative amounts of nutrients in foods and allows them to be ranked from highest to lowest. Remember, highly concentrated food such as kelp, dulse, wheat germ, and brewer's yeast is not eaten in 100-gram quantities. Therefore, they are frequently listed first, as concentrated nutrition sources. To give an idea of what 100 grams of a food represents in common measurements, the following conversions may be useful:

Approximate Equivalents

1 teaspoon fluid	=	About 5 grams
1 teaspoon dry	=	About 4 grams
1 cup milk, yogurt	=	245 grams
1 cup leafy vegetable	=	90 grams
1 cup root vegetable	=	135 grams
1 cup nuts, seeds	=	140 grams
1 cup sliced fruit	=	150 grams
1 cup cereal grain (uncooked)	=	200 grams
1 tablespoon cooking oil	=	14 grams
1 tablespoon honey molasses	=	20 grams

Carotene - Vitamin A

IU per 100 grams edible portion
(100 grams = 3-1/2 oz.)

50,500	Lamb liver	3,400	Cantaloupe
43,900	Beef liver	3,300	Butter
22,500	Calf's liver	3,300	Endive
21,600	Peppers, red chili	2,700	Apricots
		2,500	Broccoli spears
14,000	Dandelion greens	2,600	Whitefish
12,100	Chicken liver	2,000	Green onions
11,000	Carrots	1,900	Romaine lettuce
10,900	Apricots, dried	1,750	Papayas
9,300	Collard greens	1,650	Nectarines
8,900	Kale	1,600	Prunes
8,800	Sweet potatoes	1,600	Pumpkin
8,500	Parsley	1,580	Swordfish
8,100	Spinach	1,540	Cream, whipping
7,600	Turnip greens	1,330	Peaches
7,000	Mustard greens	1,200	Acorn squash
6,500	Swiss chard	1,180	Eggs
6,100	Beet greens	1,080	Chicken
5,800	Chives	1,000	Cherries, sour red
5,700	Butternut squash	970	Butterhead lettuce
4,900	Watercress	900	Asparagus
4,800	Mangos	900	Tomatoes, ripe
4,450	Peppers, sweet red	770	Peppers, green chili
4,300	Hubbard squash	690	Kidneys

640 Green peas	550 Brussels sprouts
600 Green beans	520 Okra
600 Elderberries	510 Yellow cornmeal
590 Watermelon	460 Yellow squash
580 Rutabagas	

Vitamin A from animal source foods occurs mostly as active, performed vitamin A (retinol) while that from vegetable source foods occurs as pro-vitamin A (beta-carotene and other carotenoids) which must be converted to active vitamin A by the body to be utilized. The efficiency of conversion varies among individuals; however, beta-carotene is converted more efficiently than other carotenoids. Green and deep yellow vegetables as well as deep yellow fruits are highest in beta-carotene.

Tocopherol - Vitamin E

IU per 100 grams edible portion
(100 grams = 3-1/2 oz.)

216	Wheat germ oil	18	Peanuts
90	Sunflower seeds	18	Olive oil
88	Sunflower seed oil	14	Soybean oil
72	Safflower oil	13	Peanuts, roasted
48	Almonds	11	Peanut butter
45	Sesame oil	3.6	Butter
34	Peanut oil	3.2	Spinach
29	Corn oil	3.0	Oatmeal
22	Wheat germ	3.0	Bran
		2.9	Asparagus
		2.5	Salmon

111

2.5	Brown rice	1.4	Whole-wheat bread
2.3	Rye, whole	1.0	Carrots
2.2	Rye bread, dark	.99	Peas
1.9	Pecans	.92	Walnuts
1.9	Rye & wheat crackers	.88	Bananas
		.72	Tomatoes
		.29	Lamb

Calciferol (Synthetic) - Vitamin D

IU per 100 grams edible portion
(100 grams = 3-1/2 oz.)

500	Sardines,	50	Liver
350	Salmon	50	Eggs
250	Tuna	40	Milk, fortified
150	Shrimp	40	Mushrooms
90	Butter	30	Natural cheese
90	Sunflower seeds		

Vitamin K

Micrograms (mcg) per 100 grams edible portion
(100 grams = 3-1/2 oz.)

650	Turnip greens	30	Butter
200	Broccoli	25	Pork liver
129	Lettuce	20	Oats
125	Cabbage	19	Green peas
92	Beef liver	17	Whole wheat
89	Spinach	14	Green beans
57	Watercress	11	Pork
57	Asparagus	11	Eggs
35	Cheese	10	Corn oil

8	Peaches		5	Tomatoes
7	Beef		3	Milk
7	Chicken liver		3	Potatoes
6	Raisins			

Thiamin - Vitamin B-1

Milligrams (mg) per 100 grams edible portion
(100 grams = 3-1/2 oz.)

15.61	Yeast, brewer's	.72	Wheat bran
14.01	Yeast, torula	.67	Pistachio nuts
2.01	Wheat germ	.65	Navy beans
1.96	Sunflower seeds	.63	Veal heart
1.84	Rice polishings	.60	Buckwheat
1.28	Pine nuts	.60	Oatmeal
1.14	Peanuts, with skins	.55	Whole-wheat flour
1.10	Soybeans, dry	.55	Whole-wheat
1.05	Cowpeas, dry	.51	Lamb kidneys
.98	Peanuts, without skins	.48	Lima beans, dry
.96	Brazil nuts	.46	Hazelnuts
.93	Pork, lean	.45	Lamb heart
.38	Cornmeal, whole-ground	.45	Wild rice
.86	Pecans	.43	Cashews
.85	Soybean flour	.43	Rye, whole grain
.84	Beans, pinto & red	.40	Lamb liver
.74	Split peas	.40	Lobster
.73	Millet	.38	Mung beans
		.38	Cornmeal, whole ground
		.37	Lentils
		.36	Beef kidneys

113

.35	Green peas	.24	Pumpkin & squash seeds
.34	Macadamia nuts	.23	Brains, all kinds
.34	Brown rice	.23	Chestnuts, fresh
.33	Walnuts		
.31	Garbanzos	.23	Soybean sprouts
.30	Pork liver		
.25	Garlic, cloves	.22	Peppers, red chili
.25	Beef liver		
.24	Almonds	.18	Sesame seeds, hulled
.24	Lima beans,		

Riboflavin - Vitamin B-2

Milligrams (mg) per 100 grams edible portion
(100 grams = 3-1/2 oz.)

5.06	Yeast, torula	.46	Mushrooms
4.28	Yeast, brewer's	.44	Egg yolks
		.38	Millet
3.28	Lamb liver	.36	Peppers, hot red
3.26	Beef liver		
3.03	Pork liver	.35	Soy flour
2.72	Calf's liver	.35	Wheat bran
2.55	Beef kidneys	.33	Mackerel
2.49	Chicken liver	.31	Collards
2.42	Lamb kidneys	.31	Soybeans, dry
1.36	Chicken giblets	.30	Eggs
		.29	Split peas
1.05	Veal heart	.29	Beef tongue
.92	Almonds	.26	Brains, all kinds
.88	Beef heart		
.74	Lamb heart	.26	Kale
.68	Wheat germ	.26	Parsley
.63	Wild rice	.25	Cashews

.25	Rice bran	.22	Lentils
.25	Veal	.22	Pork, lean
.24	Lamb, lean	.22	Prunes
.23	Broccoli	.22	Rye, whole grain
.23	Chicken, flesh & skin	.21	Mung beans
.23	Pine nuts	.21	Beans, pinto & red
.23	Salmon	.21	Blackeye peas
.23	Sunflower seeds	.21	Okra
.22	Navy beans	.13	Sesame seeds, hulled
.22	Beet & mustard greens		

Niacin - Vitamin B-3

Milligrams (mg) per 100 grams edible portion
(100 grams = 3-1/2 oz.)

44.4	Yeast, torula	10.7	Chicken, light meat
37.9	Yeast, brewer's	8.4	Trout
29.8	Rice bran	8.3	Halibut
28.2	Rice polishings	8.2	Mackerel
21.0	Wheat bran	8.1	Veal heart
17.2	Peanuts ,with skins	8.0	Chicken, flesh only
16.9	Lamb liver	8.0	Swordfish
16.4	Pork liver	8.0	Turkey, flesh only
15.8	Peanuts, without skins	7.7	Goose, flesh only
13.6	Beef liver	7.5	Beef heart
11.4	Calf's liver	7.2	Salmon
11.3	Turkey, light meat	6.4	Veal
10.8	Chicken liver	6.4	Beef kidneys

6.2	Wild rice	4.4	Peppers, red chili
6.1	Chicken giblets	4.4	Whole-wheat grain
5.7	Lamb, lean	4.3	Whole-wheat flour
5.6	Chicken, flesh & skin	4.2	Mushrooms
5.4	Sesame seeds	4.2	Wheat germ
5.4	Sunflower seeds	3.7	Barley
5.1	Beef, lean	3.6	Herring
5.0	Pork, lean	3.5	Almonds
4.7	Brown rice	3.2	Shrimp
4.5	Pine nuts	3.0	Haddock
4.4	Buckwheat, whole-grain	3.0	Split peas

Pantothenic Acid - a B vitamin

Milligrams (mg) per 100 grams edible portion
(100 grams = 3-1/2 oz.)

12.0	Yeast, brewer's	1.7	Soybeans
11.0	Yeast, torula	1.6	Eggs
8.0	Calf's liver	1.5	Lobster
6.0	Chicken liver	1.5	Oatmeal, dry
3.9	Beef kidneys	1.4	Buckwheat flour
2.8	Peanuts	1.4	Sunflower seeds
2.6	Brains, all kinds	1.4	Lentils
2.6	Heart	1.3	Rye flour, whole
2.2	Mushrooms	1.3	Cashews
2.0	Soybean flour	1.3	Salmon, fresh
2.0	Split peas	1.2	Camembert cheese
2.0	Beef tongue	1.2	Garbanzos
1.9	Perch	1.2	Wheat germ, toasted
1.8	Blue cheese		
1.7	Pecans		

1.2	Broccoli	1.1	Avocados
1.1	Hazelnuts	1.1	Veal, lean
1.1	Turkey, dark meat	1.0	Blackeye peas, dry
1.1	Brown rice	1.0	Wild rice
1.1	Wheat flour, whole	1.0	Cauliflower
1.1	Sardines	1.0	Chicken, dark meat
1.1	Peppers, red chili	1.0	Kale

Pyridoxine - Vitamin B-6

Milligrams (mg) per 100 grams edible portion
(100 grams = 3-1/2 oz.)

3.00	Yeast, torula	.56	Blackeye peas, dry
2.50	Yeast, brewer's		
1.25	Sunflower seeds	.56	Navy beans, dry
1.15	Wheat germ, toasted	.55	Brown rice
		.54	Hazelnuts
.90	Tuna, flesh	.54	Garbanzos, dry
.84	Beef liver	.53	Pinto beans, dry
.81	Soybeans, dry		
.75	Chicken liver	.51	Bananas
.73	Walnuts	.45	Pork, lean
.70	Salmon, flesh	.44	Albacore, flesh
.69	Trout, flesh	43	Beef, lean
.67	Calf's liver	.43	Halibut, flesh
.66	Mackerel, flesh	.43	Beef kidneys
.65	Pork liver	.42	Avocados
.63	Soybean flour	.41	Veal kidneys
.60	Lentils, dry	.34	Whole-wheat flour
.58	Lima beans, dry		
.58	Buckwheat flour	.33	Chestnuts, fresh

.30 Egg yolks
.30 Kale
.30 Rye flour
.28 Spinach
.26 Turnip greens
.26 Peppers, sweet
.25 Beef heart
.25 Potatoes
.24 Prunes
.24 Raisins
.24 Sardines
.23 Brussels sprouts
.23 Elderberries
.23 Perch, flesh
.22 Cod, flesh
.22 Barley
.22 Camembert cheese
.22 Sweet potatoes
.21 Cauliflower
.20 Popcorn, popped
.20 Red cabbage
.20 Leeks
.20 Molasses

Chapter 8

How To Ensure A Woman's Orgasm With Nutridisiacs

While a man often earns more income than his female counterpart in a family, a woman is more likely to spend the two wage earners' discretionary dollars. She spends them on food, household needs, and invests more in her own and the family's health care more regularly.

Most of the time the female member of a household does the shopping for products and services. Those services of a medical type frequently are required for correcting difficulties connected with the more complex female reproductive system. It accounts for at least 50 percent of a woman's health care complaints. This chapter will outline some common illnesses or their symptoms that affect a woman's sexuality and her ability to enjoy orgasm on a regular occurrence. According to the author Nancy Friday, over 60 percent of all American women—married or not— are nonorgasmic. They may engage in sexual intercourse but simply do not experience the climactic sensation of sexual excitement, which in

119

men occurs simultaneously with ejaculation. In women the occurrence of orgasm is much more variable, being dependent upon a number of physiological and psychological factors.

I will briefly discuss natural supplements and botanical ingredients which may be added to the family's food supply so as to relieve and possibly cure the nonorgasmic complaints connected with 10 particular discomforts or outright illnesses that affect woman. However, I won't be mentioning herbs and nutrients for easing pregnancy, labor, delivery, lactation, and other post-partum adjustments. They do affect sexuality and the ability to achieve orgasm, but they also comprise a vast arena of complications that go beyond the scope of this book. Rather, I'll focus on the ensuring that a woman achieves orgasm by having a healthy sexually responsive body through the use of nutridisiacs in foods which afford fabulous sex.

Health Conditions That Interfere with Achieving Female Orgasm

A woman's sexual woes, which may be overcome by use of nutridisiacs and other natural remedies, are classified into 10 particular causes: those related to fatigue, easy weight gain, insomnia, headache, candidiasis (the yeast syndrome), cystitis (bladder infections), menstrual difficulty, ovarian cysts, uterine fibroids, and the inevitable menopause. No woman escapes at least one of these complications involved with living in our high technology society.

The unnatural environment to which our bodies are subjected brings on any number of these 10 discomforts. For instance, 70 percent of all women living in modern industrial societies, at some time in their lives, experience vaginal yeast infections. Yeast vaginitis, in fact, provides a rich source of income for gynecologists and other primary care physicians. Premenstrual syndrome (PMS) affects a minimum of 62 percent of all adult females in North America and Europe.

Nothing described in this chapter requires that you get a doctor's prescription to use it. All of these remedies are over-the-counter, nonprescription items that you may purchase from pharmacies, natural food stores, and even some supermarkets which feature health food departments. My suggestion is that you identify what has affected your sexual ability, acquire and use the remedies which are recommended by health authorities such as herbologists, nutritionists, medical doctors, naturopaths, homeopaths, osteopaths, chiropractors, and other health care officials.

Most of the time you'll notice that dieticians are not mentioned in this text as authorities on nutridisiacs. That's because the dietician trade union is locked into the archaic information from a century ago, and this trade union forbids its members from using nutritional supplements or other items offered in <u>Foods For Fabulous Sex</u>. My observation is that the American Dietetic Association is the ultimate enemy of the holistic medical movement—a greater hindrance to the progressive use of nutrition for health care than even the American Medical Association.

Overcome Fatigue for Fabulous Sex

Fatigue is a non-specific symptom and the hallmark of many infectious or degenerative

121

diseases. Persistent fatigue for a woman may be indicative of a serious illness that requires medical attention. However, it is a complaint which warrants a course of self-care before signing up for a CT scan or some other series of sophisticated medical tests.

It is especially important to distinguish, at the onset, whether the fatigue is physiological or psychological, for if one is tired all the time engaging in sexual intercourse won't be among your priorities. "Not tonight dear, I'm just too tired" becomes a common refrain in the bedroom simply from the very real wave of fatigue that sets upon a woman.

Fatigue, the most common problem experienced by both men and women, may be associated with Chronic Fatigue Syndrome, a newly uncovered, debilitating long-term illness.

Women are more likely than men to hold more than one job, not the least of which may be parenting, so that fatigue may be present merely from the fact that too much work is attempted to be accomplished. She's just plain tired.

Also, women are more prone to anemia than men because of the monthly menstrual cycle. Anemia is a frequent cause of fatigue. With or without anemia, fatigue may come simply from a lack of good protein in the diet. This problem is particularly rampant among vegetarians. Most adults need at least 50 grams of protein daily. There are a number of excellent protein powders based on soy or milk formulas that may be taken as shakes or other drinks.

Make sure to take only sugar-free shake formulas; while sugar is a drain on the immune system and ultimately will exacerbate the fatigue. One of the typical wrong-headed ideas of traditionally practicing dieticians is that there is nothing wrong with eating products made with white crystalline sugar. Invariably you'll find, for instance, that Jello™ is part of the lunch or dinner served by dieticians in hospitals. Of course, Jello™ is about 75 percent sugar.

Another physiological cause of fatigue for a woman is endocrine imbalance, particularly low thyroid or low adrenal functioning. Hypothyroidism will be addressed in the next section, under "Easy Weight Gain." Adrenal exhaustion, of varying degrees, goes hand in hand with a stressful lifestyle. When the adrenals are constantly being stimulated by stressful jobs, relationships, deadlines, financial pressures, and other things, they start to burn out and lose the ability to respond to the environmental input. This is why stressed out people are often susceptible to inflammatory conditions such as sinus headaches, earaches, poor digestion, joint and back aches, tendinitis, and more. They get histamine reactions that result in inflammation.

The adrenals need to be nutritionally supported in order to build up again. Get the adrenals on an even keel and fatigue tends to go away so that sexual response becomes paramount again.

Herbs and Vitamins that Help Against Fatigue

Several of the most important and specific botanical sources for adrenal healing and thus sexual restoration for a female are licorice (glycerrhiza glabra), eleutherococcus, ginseng, bupleurum, and borage. Of these, licorice is the most potent for improving orgasm. The organic sugar portions (glycosides) of the dried root have a structure that is similar to the body's natural steroids.

While synthetic steroids cause glandular atrophy by giving the pituitary signals that sufficient levels of hormone are being produced, "organic" steroids such as those found in licorice nourish the endocrine system by providing the body with building blocks for regeneration.

Eleutherococcus, also known as Siberian ginseng, true ginseng (panax), and bupleurum are traditional Chinese phyto-medicinals useful for general tonifying effects and endocrine regulation. Bupleurum, are traditional Chinese phyto-medicinals useful for general tonifying effects and endocrine regulation. Bupleurum, a mild central nervous system tranquilizer, is antibiotic and enhances the immune system by decreasing histamine-induced capillary permeability.

Borage tea made from the leaves of the borage plant is known to be a gentle "mood elevator" and also acts as a restorative agent. Borage oil is a main source of gamma-linoleic acid which is efficacious for softening the lumps present in fibrocystic breast disease.

Fatigue caused by stress will usually be helped by taking a daily vitamin B complex pill which contains doses of 30 to 50 mg or so of each B vitamins.

B-1 (thiamin) changes glucose into energy or fat and prevents nervous irritability; B-2 (riboflavin) is essential in carbohydrate, fat and protein metabolism; B-3 (niacin) stimulates circulation, transports hydrogen and oxygen and is a critical cofactor in energy (ATP) production; B-5 (pantothic acid) is necessary for the production of some of the adrenal hormones; B-6 (pyridoxine) is needed for amino acid metabolism and B-12 (cyanocobalamin) is required for production of red blood cells and normal growth. In general, the B vitamins may be considered as "anti-stress" pills.

Easy Weight Gain

Easy or rapid weight gain could be a signal of a malfunctioning thyroid gland which results in insufficient output of the thyroid hormone, thyroxin. Of course, fatigue will follow but weight gain is ever present as well.

Hypothyroidism is usually accompanied by other signs of sluggish metabolism, such as cold hands and feet, puffy face, chronic hoarse voice, placid demeanor, and slow responses. Subclinical hypothyroidism is fairly common in inland states where the iodine in our country's soil has been washed out to the coasts over the centuries. The first order of treatment is to increase consumption of high-iodine foods such as **turnips, melons, lettuce, oatmeal, beets, tomatoes, and green peas.**

Avoid so-called goitrogenic foods in the brassica family, particularly cabbage. An excellent source of iodine is sea vegetables, particularly dulse and kelp. Most stores carry a variety of natural sea salt.

Clam juice, occipital and cervical spine adjustments by a chiropractor or osteopath, and thyroid glandular products are other therapeutic options to stimulate the thyroid gland. Glandulars and protomorphogens are one step below a prescription medication such as Synthroid™ and are low-heat dried, whole glands that usually come from the cow or pig without the hormone.

A much more frequent cause of easy weight gain is not exercising enough, not drinking sufficient water, and eating more calories than are being used day to day. Excess carbohydrate calories are most readily converted to fat stores.

Excess fat can often be arduous to remove. Essential fatty acids such as the omega 3 and 6 oils and the cholesterol precursors choline and inositol all help by stimulating metabolism, particularly digestion and elimination of toxins, and emulsifying the saturated fats they contact. Long sessions in low-heat saunas will literally heat fat stores and render them more liquid. The toxins which preferentially accumulate in lipids can be sweated out in this manner. It is imperative to scrub vigorously with a natural bristle brush or loofa before the fats and toxins are reabsorbed into the skin.

Insominia That Prevents Orgasm

Sleep is one of the more precious ingredients for health and vitality. Serious insomnia may come from a sleep disorder of either organic or psychological causes, and must be assessed by a medical professional.

Many of the over-the-counter plant medicines known for their sleep and relaxation-inducing qualities have a wonderful aroma. Smelling of the flowering herbs with a deep inhalation is part of the treatment known as aromatherapy. Lavender in particular is a good example of a soothing floral tea whose divine scent calms the central nervous system directly through the olfactory bulb.

Smelling is our most primordial sense; the aromatic elements penetrate into the skull and directly stimulate the olfactory bulb. Other ingredients for a bedtime floral infusion are passion flower (<u>Passiflora</u>), lime-flower (<u>Tillea</u>), lemon balm (<u>Melissa officinales</u>), skullcap (<u>Scutellaria laterifolia</u>), and verbena. All of these nonprescription botanicals are pleasant to use and do tend to induce sleep.

My recommendation is that you utilize some of the herbals mentioned in this section in order to induce a regularity in your times of sleeping. They do work, although it may take you some time to respond to them. Feeling more at ease with your body's state of relaxation, purposefully function in a sexual mode with your lover. You'll likely experience awakening stimulation from foreplay and intromission; give into these activities whole hog and let the orgasmic sensation come over you like a wave of ecstasy. It's worth the effort.

Headache As A Source Of Sexual Disturbance

Perhaps more commonly stated than fatigue as an excuse for avoiding sexual intimacy may be the alternative phrase: "Not tonight dear, I have a headache!" In fact, the prescribing and sale of headache remedies is a big money-maker in the medical and pharmaceutical businesses. A bad headache is difficult to ignore.

For practical purposes there are three major classifications of headache: the cluster headache, the tension headache, and the classic migraine.

Cluster headaches, which typically come on at the same time daily for weeks, then subside suddenly until the next round, are mostly caused by alcohol consumption.

Tension headaches are generally caused by neck and shoulder muscles that have remained rigid to bear the weight of the head (which weighs about 10 pounds) in a fixed position for hours on end. These headaches are relieved by gently rolling the neck and shoulders throughout the day, and not staring fixedly at the road, a TV, computer screen or desk work for more than 20 minutes at a time.

Massage helps a lot. In terms of nutritional supplements for tension headache, the natural mineral muscle relaxants work well, especially if taken in the evening. A good multivitamin/mineral supplement would contain about 500 mg of calcium, 300 mg of magnesium, and 100 mg of potassium, preferably in the citrate or ascorbate form.

Phytomedicinals, also referred to as "herbs" for tension headache include skullcap, passion flower, hops (Humulus lupulus), henbane (Hyoscyamus ruger), and the exotic herb Jamaican dogwood (Piscidiaerythrina). Women taking these herbs for headache relief will be pleasantly surprised at their nontoxic effectiveness. Sometimes they work better than aspirin and without the stomach-burning side effects.

Migraine is a complex and often refractory problem. People are well advised to avoid any identified allergens and high-tyramine sources such as the drinking of red wine or eating aged cheeses, pickled or cured meats, bananas, avocados, broad beans, and fermented or yeast-containing foods. They should avoid additionally basking in bright sunlight, stress, feeling resentment, or taking drugs and caffeine (such as coffee). A moderate dose, from 100 to 300 mg of niacin at the onset of the migraine during the "aura" or "halo lights" phase may avert the pounding sequel of pain.

Botanicals that are known to help migraine include peppermint (<u>Mentha</u> <u>piperita</u>), ginger (<u>Zingiber</u> <u>officinale</u>), and "old man's beard" (<u>Usnea</u> <u>barbata</u>).

A number of victims get relief from headaches by self-administering a cool enema. A sturdy douche-bag can double as a hot water bottle for holding the enema fluid. Hydrocollators, epsom salt soaks, and ice packs all can be helpful in reducing the frequency of headaches when they are applied periodically. Getting rid of your headache before it's anticipated to strike is the way to achieve orgasmic response through sexual contact with the person you love.

Candidiasis and Other Yeast Infections

<u>Candida</u> <u>albicans</u> is the scientific name of a fungus which naturally inhabits, in a controlled quantity, the human intestinal tract. It does not belong in the vagina. It most certainly does not belong in the blood stream. In our bodies, which are altered and made to adapt (but inadequately) to our industrialized society, <u>C.</u> <u>albicans</u> does abnormally invade both of these abnormal regions and does play havoc in them.

Candida, like all fungi, loves sugar. Sugared foods of any type stimulate the fungus to overgrow and create that series of disturbing signs and symptoms (including vaginal discharge) known as the yeast syndrome.

One of the most effective agents in combating this yeast overgrowth and other nonspecific vaginal yeast infections is tannic acid. The tannins, which were originally used to cure animal skins into hides, bind to the yeast and prevent it from attaching to the host's mucous membranes in the gut and the vagina. Black tea, witch hazel (Hamamelis virginiana) and golden seal (Hydrastis canadensis) are all high in tannins and have proven themselves effective for controlling the yeast syndrome.

Golden seal is also an excellent source of berberine, which is extremely healing to all mucosal surfaces, from mouth to anus, and including the interstitial alveoli (those spaces between lung cells), bladder, and vagina.

Besides too much sugar intake, another cause of yeast syndrome complications is an altered mucosal pH. Many vaginal yeast infections are associated with reduced acidity, or too much alkaline an environment. The vagina needs to be somewhat acidic to stay healthy. Ejaculated semen which contains sperm is very alkaline. Periodic douching with restorative botanicals is advisable, particularly when entertaining a new consort or engaging in sex with your spouse. A simple boric acid douche very effectively restores optimal vaginal pH. A good formula for you to use as a restorative douche might include comfrey (Symphytum officinale) for its epithelium-repairing properties, old man's beard for its anti-viral properties, and yarrow (Achillea millefolium) for its anti-inflammatory action, all in a solution of diluted white vinegar.

The Bladder Infections of Cystitis

Sexual activity is frequently the cause of strange, warm, fuzzy bacteria winding their way into the urethra and up into the bladder. Your bladder is usually a sterile environment where said bacteria indulge in replication. If you are not used to having an invasion by these new, warm, fuzzy bacteria, you'll experience the condition euphemistically referred to as "honeymoon" cystitis, even though you are not on your honeymoon.

Cranberry juice of the unsweetened type really does work to rid a woman of this problem. Cranberries work not so much because they acidify the urinary tract which ordinarily helps to keep the bacterial population down to a dull roar, but because the berries contain various ingredients which form complexes with the bacteria. These complexes prevent them from adhering to the walls of the bladder and urethra. Drinking plenty of water then flushes the critter-complexes out through urination.

Plant medicines useful for cystitis include all berberine-containing species such as buchu, golden seal, and oregon grape root. Also working well are bearberry (Uva ursi) which has been used successfully since antiquity to soothe, tone, and strengthen the urinary system, dandelion (Taraxacum officinale), a diuretic, horsetail (Equisetum arvense) for cellular repair, thyme (Thymus vulgaris) which is antiseptic, and juniper (Juniperus communis) which is contraindicated with concomitant kidney involvement. It's practically a certainty that eliminating cystitis from your life will bring you much closer to satisfying sex and its subsequent enduring orgasm.

PMS and Other Menstrual Difficulties

As discussed in Chapter 4, the incidence of premenstrual syndrome has increased in recent decades with greater environmental stressors, including hormones and pesticides in the food chain. PMS symptoms typically occur during the luteal phase of the menstrual cycle, from ovulation to the onset of menses, and may be generally categorized in four symptomatic clusters: anxiety, bloating, cravings and depression. Most women experience a combination of these symptoms. Assuredly the annoying symptoms remove any feelings of sexuality and are major obstacles to orgasmic bliss.

Vitamins and minerals in supplement form or from the foods listed in Chapter 7 do help overcome PMS. Nutritional supplements should be tailored to the specific symptoms, but generally may include vitamins B-6, folic acid, and the mineral magnesium throughout the month.

Some of the most popular "female" herbs include red raspberry leaf (Rubus idaeus) of the organic type because commercial Rubus tends to be heavily fumigated; wild or Mexican yam (Dioscorea villosa), Siberian ginseng, squaw vine (Mitchella repens), chaste-tree (Vitex agnus-castus), dandelion which is a potassium-sparing diuretic for bloating as well as a liver cleanser because it conjugates the excess estrogens and allows for rapid excretion, and dong quai (Angelica sinensis) known as the woman's ginseng.

In Chinese medicine the uterus is thought to be an organ that dislikes "cold" and therefore warming herbs such as cinnamon and ginger and warming foods such as garlic and onions, provide relief.

Menstrual cramping, by contrast, generally happens during the first days of menstruation, because of blood clots being pushed through the muscular cervix. Menstrual cramps can be ameliorated by beginning an increased course of calcium/magnesium 10 days before onset of menses, taken in the evening away from vitamin C which tends to chelate minerals. Herbal formulations for cramps are best based around the cohosh roots, in particular black cohosh (<u>Cimicifuga</u> <u>racemosa</u>), blue cohosh (<u>Caulophyllum</u> <u>thalictroides</u>), cramp bark (<u>Viumum</u> <u>opulus</u>) and various nervines such as skullcap and valerian root.

Ovarian Cysts

From estrogen-ripening-eggs in the ovary (almost always switching in their ripening pattern from left to right on alternate months), ovarian cysts may develop. When the egg cannot ripen quite enough to burst through the ovarian wall, after which it typically floats up into the fallopian tubes, it stretches and grows while remaining attached to the ovary.

Useful vitamin and mineral nutrients include A, E, C, and B-complex, and zinc. There is an exceptionally useful herbal formulation, named after an old-timer naturopathic physician, Dr. Turska, based on the combination of botanicals monkshood (<u>Aconitum</u> <u>napellus</u>), yellow jasmine (<u>Gelsemium</u> <u>sempervirens</u>), wild hops or clinging vine (<u>Bryonia</u>) and poke root (<u>Phytolacca</u> <u>americanum</u>).

Plant medicine that balance the hormones, so-called phyto-estrogens, are useful here, as with many female complaints. Alfalfa (Medicago sativa) is a readily available and potent example of a phyto-estrogen plant.

If you have ovarian cysts, I advise you avoid ingesting dairy products since they tend to stimulate their formation.

Uterine Fibroids

In medical language this condition of uterine fibroids is called leiomyoma, and is the most common benign tumor in women. It is one of the excuses for hysterectomy—the surgical removal of the uterus, and sometimes also of the ovaries. Hysterectomy should not be undertaken lightly, for this organ has a structural function in preventing prolapse of the other abdominal organs even if not functioning for reproduction purposes.

Uterine fibroids are considerably more difficult to treat than ovarian cysts, especially if they are embedded in the uterine musculature. Before surgery, women may want to attempt a therapeutic combination of the lover's diet described in my early chapters, exercise, and botanicals. The basic idea is to decease exogenous estrogen from eating meats, chicken, eggs, and dairy products and help the liver clear out endogenous estrogens. Removing allergens and sources of inflammation, particularly red meat and dairy products from the diet is essential.

Exercise as with the device developed by the Association for Cardiovascular Therapies described in Chapter 6, the Sexersizer, increases blood circulation to the pelvic area and its associated

134

genitals. It is most useful for overcoming and then preventing fibroid tumors in the uterus.

Alternating hot and cold sitz baths are equally stimulating to the pelvic area. Liver cleansing herbs such as dandelion and milk thistle (<u>Silybum</u> <u>marianum</u>) are excellent for clearing out accumulated hormones and toxins. A tincture of pasque flower (<u>Pulsatilla</u> <u>vulgaris</u>) may help decrease fibroids, too. In other words, the way to restore healthy pelvic organs is to approach treatment holistically, without drugs and with lots of attention to yourself.

The Inevitable Menopause

As discussed in detail in Chapter 3, the normal cessation of menstruation which typically begins around age 50. Many women, contrary to popular belief, rejoice in this freedom from real or perceived reproductive obligation, and come into their full creative power at this time.

Nutrition with certain food supplements is exceptionally helpful here. Vitamin D, vitamin E, magnesium, calcium, inositol, B-complex, chromium, and selenium are all helpful for restoring the female genitals' sexual capacity during and following menopause.

Nutritional self-therapy provides many options from vegetarian diet to symptom-specific supplements. **Beet greens,** for instance, are both exceptionally rich in minerals and vitamins and lipotropic—liver cleansing.

Sage (Salvia officinalis) works well for hot flashes, as does the combination of vitex, blue cohosh, fennel, licorice, and angelica. Ginseng is excellent for vaginal dryness. Licorice potentates the remaining estrogen, which may allow for the decision not to use synthetic estrogen replacement. The major argument for estrogen replacement therapy (ERT) is the prevention of osteoporosis. But maintaining bone health with nutrients that are specific for bone growth is another, perhaps more direct, option. It also avoids the complication of increased risk for breast and uterine cancer.

So you do have the nutritional means of conquering symptoms and signs of illnesses which interfere with a woman's ability to perform in bed and enjoy herself in the process. Nutridisiacs of the types described in this chapter will do the job for you if you act on information that you've been given. A woman's libido may be elevated, but her genitals face obstacles because of yeast, PMS, cystitis, menopause, or some other physical problem. Do try the nutritional techniques available to you so that orgasmic paradise may be yours once again.

Chapter 9

Overcoming Impotence

Fear of the unknown is perhaps the greatest of all the fears that trouble mankind. This is why it is so very important to understand what impotence is and what may cause it.

You must realize that your sexual ability cannot just "go away" mysteriously. Sex itself is so often misunderstood that many men—yes, the vast majority—think that potency is some kind of magic talent. Well, it's not magic...it's a physical fact. And, so, therefore, is impotence.

Impotence happens for a reason—whether it be emotional or physical or a combination of the two. Furthermore, the inability to have an erection happens to every man at one time or another.

So, let's understand three facts right from the beginning.

1) Impotence is common
2) Impotence is temporary
3) Impotence is curable

Impotence is nothing more than the reduced or absent ability to get and maintain an erection of the penis hard enough to insert into the female.

Primarily, it has to do with the penis, not the entire man who owns it. It has to do with erection ability and nothing else. Remember that the vast majority of men troubled with impotence are active, strong, alert and effective in every other way. They are men through and through.

At some time or other in life everyone goes through some form of illness. Similarly, at least once in a lifetime just about everyone gets a sexual problem. It is wrong for the man with impotence to think of himself as alone, or as one of a tiny minority of suffering victims. There are less than a dozen classes of sex problems shared between the whole population of the Earth. So it follows that at any time an awful lot of men have impotence. Indeed, if we regard it as a disease (and strictly speaking anything that disturbs the 'ease' must be 'disease') it is probably the most common of all 'diseases' in Western Society today.

Impotence should always be regarded as a purely temporary condition. Unfortunately with some men, the things that cause the trouble keep on happening. So, impotence keeps on and on being temporary. In other words, it looks permanent. But it isn't.

The main object here is to assemble all the successful methods of treating impotence and converge them into one overall regime, to overwhelm the problem with such a high and confident cure rate that for almost everyone the problem will be improved or solved. But, in order to put an end to impotence, it is necessary to understand the sheer mechanics of sexual function.

Several parts of the body are involved in erection. Primarily, sexual excitement takes place in the brain. It is to this central control point that the body's nerves bring sexually provocative messages. The images from the eyes, the scent of perfumes and body odors, the sounds of affectionate words, or romantic music, the touching and being touched anywhere on the body, all these sensations are racing through the circuitry of the brain and are being mixed in with other things like sexual memories and preferences. Some of the glands like the pituitary, the adrenals and the testicles produce hormones that all fit into the excitement pattern. Eventually, through the nerves of the spinal cord and the sympathetic nervous system, messages reach the penis and blood pumps swiftly into its spongy tissue spaces. At the same time, small muscles around the root of the penis contract to stop the blood from getting back into the body. The result is that more blood goes into the penis than gets out and, like a balloon filling with air, the penis swells and stiffens. The things to remember are that several parts of the body are essential to the erection process, but that the two key points are the brain sending out the sexual instructions and the penis muscles contracting to retain blood.

When something goes wrong with the mechanism, and it need only occur at one spot to disrupt the whole process, then the penis stubbornly refuses to become erect and remains too soft to get into the vagina. That is impotence.

There are probably as many causes of impotence as there are men on this planet...but these causes break down into a few broad categories that cover 95 percent of men.

Aging

It is true that sexual power does seem to decline as the years roll by, but the decrease is not very big or significant. A man, otherwise fit and healthy, should not experience an unwanted decrease of libido of more than about 10 percent by the age of 60 and another 10 percent by 70. However, the frequency of his erections and their strength does diminish. Furthermore, whereas in his earlier years, just to look at his partner produced an erection, increasingly after the age of 40 he is likely to need more actual direct attention (stroking, playing, etc.) to the penis itself to achieve the same result. This is normal. It is sad and wrong that it is sometimes a source of dismay to his partner who mistakes it for a declining interest in her or a reduction of her own sexual attraction and ability.

In addition, there is a social misconception about sexual behavior in older people. Our society for some false reason or other has a tendency to think that sex between older people is rather nasty, dirty, unhygienic and so on. This may well arise from the way people seem to think of their parents having sexual connections as a pretty unwholesome business. It isn't true. Good sex is good for everyone. Be that as it may, there is a conditioned idea that one ought to refrain from sex as one gets older. This is totally untrue too, but just the idea can cause potency problems.

Obesity

Being overweight can play havoc with your hormones. It can make your circulation more sluggish, even push your blood pressure up to dangerous extremes. All these things can make it difficult for you to perform.

Plus, that excess weight may make it difficult for your penis to protrude adequately from your body. Or, you may feel embarrassed about your body to the point that your impotence is a defense mechanism.

Drugs

Prescription medicines, alcohol and even the use of illegal drugs such as marijuana and cocaine have been implicated in a vast number of impotence cases. These drugs cause impotence by interrupting the chain of mechanisms that create erection. Some of the tablets given for emotional depression are culprits, and so are some treatments for blood pressure. If you suspect such a cause, then discuss it with your doctor. He may well be able to prescribe for you a more suitable medication. In this sense, alcohol is also a drug. A little may make you perform better. A lot is sure to cause disaster. Very few drunken men fail to suffer from impotence.

Diseases

There are literally dozens of diseases that count impotence as one of their symptoms. Diabetes, heart disease, prostatitis, Alzheimer's, cirrhosis of the liver and kidney disease to name a few.

Regardless of severity of the disease, if a man wishes to function sexually, he should be able to. There are numerous ways to contend with this, including surgery and medical intervention.

Fatigue

Simply being too tired happens to everyone some days. But it can go on and on if one or both partners are caught in a hectic lifestyle that means always being too tired. Such a couple has its priorities all wrong. I described fatigue for a female and what happens to her orgasmic response in Chapter 8.

Boredom

This is one of the easiest potency pitfalls to overcome. An otherwise happy couple may feel after being together for many years they've explored everything there is about sex. Sex has been the same pattern for so long it's no longer an excitement. They may not be too worried about this. But some will feel it's worth looking for new and more inventive factors in the flagging sex life.

Emotional Problems

This is perhaps the largest and most crippling group of impotence causes.

It is unfortunate that in illness or reduced efficiency of all kinds, sexual performance is immediately dispensable. So it is with all emotional illnesses or 'diseases'. Stress, especially of a severe or continuous nature, affects the brain function. So does anxiety. So does depression. So does mere unhappiness. So do those mentally injurious incidents from earlier life, repressed and forgotten by the conscious mind but stored deep in the memory banks. Some are so full of unresolved emotion that they exert their influence even at times of unconnected excitement. Being in debt, being overworked, too much competition in the rat-race, all of these have a powerful, negative effect on potency.

But, let me give you a few instances of real emotional trouble. Keep in mind that I'm not asking you to play amateur psychologist. However, I want you to realize that the mind exerts a powerful influence over your penile powers. The interesting thing is, though, that a few simple mental and physical exercises can overcome even the most stubborn and complex mental hang-ups.

For example, a common cause of impotence is sexual fright caused by childhood sex fears. The wet or sexual dream frightens some men who think it results from childhood sex irregularities or from defective organs. Any of these beliefs can cause impotence. In such cases, the man is convinced that he can't engage in satisfactory sexual relations, especially if beginning attempts aren't too successful. It may help allay a man's fears when he learns that wet dreams are a natural function by which the seed sacs are emptied automatically when regular evacuation is not possible.

Masturbation is another major cause of sexual fear. Many men blame that former indulgence for their present difficulty to engage in intercourse. Masturbation shouldn't cause such difficulty. It is a natural stage through which almost all boys and girls go, and if it did cause impotence, practically every man would be impotent and every woman frigid. The real trouble lies in that masturbation creates in some men a sense of guilt or shame and it is this factor of guilt that contributes to impotence.

Many men lose their ability to perform satisfactory coitus because they brood over the length of their penis, or to be more exact, the lack of length. The size of the penis, either in the flaccid or erect state, has no effect on the performance of coitus. The ability to maintain erection is the important function of the penis. Despite the size of your organ, however, with the adoption of a suitable position, almost all men should be capable of satisfactory sexual relations with their partners.

A subspecialty of psychotherapy, sex therapy attempts to identify and remove the destructive attitudes responsible for the patient's dysfunction and improve the sexual response. Taking several forms, the discipline includes sex counseling to deal with a big or little crisis, education to separate myth from reality, and correction to help the client or couple adopt new beliefs and attitudes about themselves. Insight therapy and behavior modification are also used.

But sex therapy may not be successful. The practice has grown little outside the Masters and Johnson model, which doesn't do much to encourage personal breakthroughs or insights. Also, seldom is medical and surgical treatment instituted for true physiological problems. If actual physical impairment is causing the impotence, a sex therapist often washes his or her hands of the patient and referral may or may not be made for such necessary treatment. Sex therapists hardly ever consider using proven nutritional repair, acupuncture, diet control, hypnotism, or other holistic techniques. A medical work-up may be ordered but it seldom is followed up, since many sex therapists remain convinced that dysfunction is largely a psychogenic problem.

A mental factor very often overlooked is that a man may become impotent because he has ceased to love his wife and intercourse may actually be repugnant to him, even though he may not know it. His subconscious lack of love is thus manifested by unsatisfactory (undesired) coitus. Or the man may be in love with some other woman. He may not be conscious of this, either, but this will subconsciously prevent him from satisfactorily engaging his wife in intercourse. This, too, may be a problem for a doctor or psychiatrist to unravel.

Medications and Miscellaneous

There are numerous prescription drugs and physical ailments that can cause impotence. This is why I suggest that any man suffering from impotence should go to see his doctor.

However, regaining your potency means regaining command of your body. I stress: you must be well informed about how your body functions.

Indeed, the list of illnesses that include impotence as one of their symptoms is long. But, the most important thing to remember is this: no matter what the cause, 98 percent of all impotent men can find a cure of one kind or another.

Not only do illnesses cause impotence, but so do the drugs that treat the illnesses. According to Dr. John Morley, a professor at the University of California at Los Angeles, "Medications have been considered to be responsible for impotence in up to 25 percent of the cases." He emphasized that the problem was especially severe for those using drugs to combat hypertension.

I'm sure that these long lists of things associated with impotence may be somewhat alarming. Actually, they should make you feel better—because for each one there is a solution, often a simple solution. The point is, you must stop blaming yourself for your sexual problems. A potency problem, no matter how severe, can never be blamed on oneself. In fact, blame and guilt are often themselves primary causes of impotence.

As I said earlier, regaining your sex life is something that you really can do on your own with the help of nutridisiacs. Certainly, if you wish, you may see a counselor or sexual therapist for your problems. Self exploration and understanding are sure to follow.

So, we can see that some problems are genetic, some societal and some personal. But with proper knowledge you can begin to deal with basic potency problems and succeed, especially if you eat certain foods described in the previous chapters.

Chapter 10

Your Personal Potential Guide:

Tests for Sexual and Lifestyle Stress

This is a chapter that most people find fun and enlightening. The tests will help you determine your stress load, and are simply meant to be informative and are not to be construed as medical diagnoses.

A stress test that is commonly used to determine long-term stress is the Life Events Scale developed by Thomas Holmes and Richard Rahe. Circle the point values of the events that apply to you, then check to see if your total point score falls into the low, moderate, or high stress-symptom-risk range. This will give you some idea of where your long-term stresses lie at the moment, and how much of an impact stress may have had on your life in the past year.

Life Event	Point Value
Death of a spouse	100
Divorce	73
Marital separation	65
Jail Term	63

Death of close family member	63
Personal injury or illness	53
Marriage	50
Fired at work	47
Marital reconciliation	45
Retirement	44
Change in health of family member	44
Pregnancy	40
Sex difficulties	39
Gain of new family member	39
Business readjustment	39
Change in financial state	38
Death of close friend	37
Change to different line of work	36
Change in number of arguments with spouse	35
Mortgage or loan over $10,000	31
Foreclosure of mortgage or loan	30
Change in responsibilities at work	29
Son or daughter leaving home	29
Trouble with in-laws	29
Outstanding personal achievement	28
Spouse begin or stop work	26
Begin or end school	26
Change in living conditions	25
Revision of personal habits	24
Trouble with boss	23
Change in work hours or conditions	20
Change in residence	20
Change in schools	20
Change in recreation	19
Change in church activities	19
Change in social activities	18
Mortgage or loan less than $10,000	17
Change in sleeping habits	16
Change in number of family get-togethers	15
Change in eating habits	15
Vacation	13

Christmas	12
Minor violations of the law	11

Your Total: _____

In their studies, Homes and Rahe found that people with scores over 300 points for one year had an 80 percent risk of becoming seriously ill or vulnerable to depression during the following year. Those with scores between 200 and 300 points had a 50 percent, or moderate, risk. Although these figures cannot accurately predict the risk for any particular individual, they do confirm the correlation between life-change stress and both physical and emotional health. Furthermore, if you are a Type A or Type A+ person, you are potentially at higher risk for stress symptoms than a person who practices Type B behavior patterns.

So, let us next find out if you have any symptoms of the high-stress type A personality. Answer yes, no or sometimes to the following questions and add up your score.

1)   I can never be satisfied with my achievements.

_____ yes   _____ no   _____ sometimes

2)   I am always impatient with myself.

_____ yes   _____ no   _____ sometimes

3)   I am always impatient with others (but try to hide it).

_____ yes   _____ no   _____ sometimes

4) I tend to over schedule myself to the point that one traffic jam throws my whole day off.

_____ yes _____ no _____ sometimes

5) I prefer too much to do to too little to do.

_____ yes _____ no _____ sometimes

6) I work better under pressure, so I often let projects pile up until I am under the gun.

_____ yes _____ no _____ sometimes

7) I am openly competitive at sports, but at work I secretly assess other's progress and then expect even more of myself.

_____ yes _____ no _____ sometimes

8) I expect so much of myself that I cannot tolerate any further demands or criticism.

_____ yes _____ no _____ sometimes

9) I experience telephone anxiety. Every ringing telephone represents a new problem for me to solve.

_____ yes _____ no _____ sometimes

10) I hate to wait!

_____ yes _____ no _____ sometimes

11) I have a quick temper, which I try to hide.

_____ yes   _____ no   _____ sometimes

12) I do not feel that I am really lovable, so work becomes my world.

_____ yes   _____ no   _____ sometimes

13) I cannot control my family's feelings, so work becomes my world.

_____ yes   _____ no   _____ sometimes

14) I have "status" insecurity, so work becomes my world.

_____ yes   _____ no   _____ sometimes

Count up each yes vote as 3 points, each sometimes as 1 point and each no as 0 points.

30 to 42 points - extreme stress, Type A+
15 to 29 points - high stress, Type A
7 to 15 points - moderate stress, Type A/B
below 7 points - lower stress, Type B

Being a Type A or A+ doesn't have to be a permanent thing. If you intellectually realize that being driven is a negative, then you can make a conscious effort to change yourself. Let's learn a few positives from the lower stress Type B personality.

A Type B person:

- is not as stressed by setbacks or failures, since expectations for themselves and for life are more realistic than optimistic.

- is not as obsessed by past glories or future fantasies, since they accept who they are today, rather than focusing on who they were yesterday or who they should be tomorrow.

- is not as impatient when they delegate responsibility, since they are less competitive than a Type A and less likely to personalize others' behaviors.

- is not a perfectionistic, since they have a greater sense of security, and is not as approval-seeking, since they have a greater sense of self-esteem.

- doesn't over schedule themselves as often, since they are more likely to do what they can do rather than to try to do what they think they should do.

- is not self-conscious about playing, dancing, chancing something new, or laughing out loud, since they are not monitoring their behavior for "appearances."

- is not as apt to have trouble giving and receiving affection and compliments, since they have less general hostility.

As you can see the Type B man or woman is able to enjoy life to a greater degree than the Type A. The Type B man or woman is also less likely to suffer from impotence and marital/sexual stress. This brings us to a couple of tests that are quite revealing. Let's begin with the:

MARITAL STRESS TEST

I am least tolerant of behaviors of my spouse or children that I dislike in myself.
_____ True _____ False

I often feel jealous or suspicious of my spouse after I've had a fantasy about being unfaithful.
_____ True _____ False

I feel at a loss when my spouse or children are upset.
_____ True _____ False

I find that I am often annoyed at my spouse or children for no reason.
_____ True _____ False

I suspect that I use my family as scapegoats for daily tension buildup.
_____ True _____ False

I act unemotional even when I don't feel that way.
_____ True _____ False

I feel so guilty after being angry at my spouse or children that I make up to them by being overindulgent.
_____ True _____ False

I see my spouse and children as extensions of me, and expect them to behave as I would behave.
_____ True _____ False

I often feel defensive, like I am "walking on eggs", when I am home.
_____ True _____ False

I find that I avoid going home by doing extra work at the office.
_____ True _____ False

I feel that I am not appreciated by my spouse or family.
_____ True _____ False

I eat/smoke/drink compulsively when I come home at night.
_____ True _____ False

I have lost interest in being intimate or sexual with my spouse.
_____ True _____ False

I frequently fall asleep and/or awaken earlier than I would like.
_____ True _____ False

I fear that I may become physically violent at home.
_____ True _____ False

I find it hard to think clearly when I am at home.
_____ True _____ False

I seem to have no sense of humor when I am at home.
_____ True _____ False

I feel like I am "trapped" in my marriage.
_____ True _____ False

I feel lonely when I am with my spouse and/or family.
_____ True _____ False

If you checked off any of these statements as true, you have a good deal of introspection to do. Should you answer True to any of the last 10 questions, you may want to consider seeking the help of a marital counselor for both you and your spouse. These are more serious indications of trouble in the marriage.

The next test goes directly to the heart of the issue: your sexual ability. Even one check mark means that you need help.

[ ] Never able to get an erection.
[ ] Cannot experience orgasm.
[ ] Too tired to start or finish sex act.
[ ] Desire sex but cannot perform.
[ ] Lack of sexual aggression and confidence.
[ ] Erections fail in specific circumstances.
[ ] Erection doesn't last long enough.

Now that you know there's a good chance that your sexual problems may be caused by your mental attitude, I suggest that you check off the words that apply to the way you feel about sex. Be honest.

Whenever I attempt sex, have sex or think about sex, I sometimes feel...

[ ] Intimidated   [ ] Frail
[ ] Uncertain   [ ] Incapable
[ ] Bored   [ ] Insecure
[ ] Dirty   [ ] Shaky
[ ] Resentful   [ ] Unable
[ ] Tired   [ ] Unsound
[ ] Disinterested   [ ] Stupid
[ ] Cautious   [ ] Crippled
[ ] Cowardly   [ ] Exhausted
[ ] Disabled   [ ] Helpless
[ ] Harmless   [ ] Ineffective
[ ] Incompetent   [ ] Powerless
[ ] Meek   [ ] Small
[ ] Sickly   [ ] Unfit
[ ] Useless   [ ] Vulnerable
[ ] Defective   [ ] Comic
[ ] Exposed   [ ] Frustrated
[ ] Impotent   [ ] Rejected
[ ] Inept   [ ] Anemic
[ ] Puny   [ ] Deficient
[ ] Strengthless   [ ] Fragile
[ ] Unimportant   [ ] Inadequate
[ ] Weak   [ ] Inferior
[ ] Broken   [ ] Shaken
[ ] Demoralized   [ ] Trivial
[ ] Misunderstood   [ ] Unqualified

If eight or more of these words were meaningful to you, your lack of sexual achievement may be psychological. At the very least, your sex life is not the joyous, explosive experience it should be.

But, take heart, by following the recipies and information in this therapeutic guide you will absolutely rejuvenate your sexual potency and you'll discover the many ways that <u>Foods For Fabulous Sex</u> can change your life.

Summary

The substances that medical science is willing to label as nutridisiacs are few and far between. This doesn't mean, however, that there is a shortage of substances. On the contrary, dozens of substances such as histamine, niacin, L-dopa, parachlorophenylalanine, garlic and L-tryptophan are currently being tested for their penile powers. But medical science is slow and cautious. This is why I suggest that, when it comes to aphrodisiac substances, you limit your repertoire to those ingredients with a clean bill of health.

The best advice that I can offer to people who wish to enjoy the benefits of any nutridisiac is to a) maintain a healthy body in an atmosphere that is as low in stress as possible, b) use only the highest quality herbal and natural substances to spark romance and renewed interest, and c) keep in mind that sometimes charisma is all a substance— or a man—needs to produce an erection or a woman to attain an orgasm.

Fabulous sex is much more than pulsating with pleasure. It's a way of looking at life. A way of taking command of one's self and one's environment.

You have been given the gift of sexual enjoyment. If you now know how to visualize taking charge of your life, pleasure and potency are yours just for the taking.

Keep in mind that if you're ready for supreme potency, fabulous sex will be ready for you. Keep this manual handy. The techniques and instructions on sexual matters should always be referred to. Don't delay. A rich and full life of sexual pleasures and success is waiting!